Advance Praise for *So What Can I Eat?!*

"In *So What Can I Eat?!* Elisa explains the latest nutritional guidelines in an upbeat and encouraging tone and using a good commonsense approach. For those who want to change their food and fitness habits for the better, this book is priceless!"

—Solomon Katz, Ph.D., director of the Krogman Center for Childhood Growth and Development at the University of Pennsylvania and editor in chief, Scribner's *Encyclopedia of Food and Culture*

"This book is fabulous! Elisa reveals how eating healthfully can be a reality for everyone. She guides readers through the process of evaluating their own dietary and lifestyle behaviors and making realistic changes based on sound science. Best of all, Elisa's genuine and positive approach makes the book relatable, accessible, and encouraging for all readers!"

—Lyssie Lakatos, R.D., C.D.N., and Tammy Lakatos Shames, R.D., C.D.N., authors of *Fire Up Your Metabolism: 9 Proven Principles for Burning Fat and Losing Weight Forever*

"Elisa captures the essence of the Dietary Guidelines to help consumers follow eating plans that are helpful, healthy, and delicious! Her practical tips and recipes provide a sensible and scientific approach to eating right and staying fit."

—Judith A. Gilbride, Ph.D., R.D., F.A.D.A., chair of New York University's Department of Nutrition, Food Studies, and Public Health

"*So What Can I Eat?!* presents an upbeat and user-friendly guide to understanding the current federal nutrition guidelines. I highly recommend it."

—Lisa R. Young, Ph.D., R.D., adjunct assistant professor, New York University, and author of *The Portion Teller: Smartsize Your Way to Permanent Weight Loss*

"This book is a great option for those who are tired of fad diets and ready to adopt a sensible approach to healthy eating. Elisa's passion for sharing her professional and personal knowledge with others makes *So What Can I Eat?!* an inspiring, enjoyable read."

—Cynthia Sass, M.P.H., M.A., R.D., author of *Your Diet Is Driving Me Crazy*

So What *Can* I Eat?!

How to Make Sense
of the New
Dietary Guidelines
for Americans
and Make Them
Your Own

ELISA ZIED, M.S., R.D., C.D.N.,
WITH RUTH WINTER, M.S.

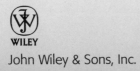

WILEY

John Wiley & Sons, Inc.

Published by John Wiley & Sons, Inc., Hoboken, New Jersey
Published simultaneously in Canada

Design and composition by Navta Associates, Inc.

The information contained in this book is not intended to serve as a replacement for professional medical advice. Any use of the information in this book is at the reader's discretion. The author and the publisher specifically disclaim any and all liability arising directly or indirectly from the use or application of any information contained in this book. A health care professional should be consulted regarding your specific situation.

For general information about our other products and services, please contact our Customer Care Department within the United States at (800) 762-2974, outside the United States at (317) 572-3993 or fax (317) 572-4002.

Wiley also publishes its books in a variety of electronic formats. Some content that appears in print may not be available in electronic books. For more information about Wiley products, visit our web site at www.wiley.com.

Library of Congress Cataloging-in-Publication Data:

Zied, Elisa.
    So what can I eat?! : how to make sense of the new dietary guidelines for Amer-icans and make them your own / Elisa Zied and Ruth Winter.
        p. cm.
    Includes index.
    ISBN-13 978-0-471-77201-9 (pbk.)
    ISBN-10 0-471-77201-1 (pbk.)
    1. Nutrition policy—United States. 2. Nutrition. 3. Food. I. Winter, Ruth, 1930–II. Title.
    TX360.U6Z54 2006
    363.8'5610973—dc22

Printed in the United States of America

10 9 8 7 6 5 4 3 2 1

To my wonderful husband, Brian, and our
two precious boys, Spencer and Eli

Contents

Acknowledgments

There are so many wonderful people I have to thank for helping me create this book: my literary agent, Stacey Glick, for her enthusiastic guidance and support; my editor, Teryn Johnson, my production editor, Lisa Burstiner, and all the people at John Wiley & Sons who put this book together so masterfully; and Mike Morgan, for a bright and cheerful cover photo. Last but not least, I'd like to thank Ruth Winter, my collaborator, for her wit, wisdom, and constant encouragement throughout the book-writing process.

I thank my friends and colleagues who reviewed parts of the manuscript and provided helpful suggestions and many of the delicious homemade recipes featured in this book: Maria "Linda" Arevalo, Keri Gans, Dave Grotto, Harvey Herman, Halee Hochman, Randi Odesser, Alex Rafal, Anne Sailer, Cynthia Sass, Barbara Sickmen, Ron Sickmen, Carolyn Siden, and Linda Stegman. A big thank-you goes out to the many talented people who reviewed and tested the recipes in this book: Ron Greitzer, Claudia Sidoti, Amy Marcus, Gwynn Mueller, and Jill Sloane.

I'd also like to thank the incredible public relations team at the American Dietetic Association for the opportunity to fulfill one of my professional dreams. Doris Acosta, Kelly Liebbe, Irene Perconti, Tom Ryan, Liz Spittler, and last but not least, the wonderful Lori Ferme make it a pleasure for me to be a part of this amazing organization. I'd also like to thank my fellow ADA spokespeople. I am humbled to be a part of this dynamic and amazing group of individuals.

A very special thank-you goes to two of my mentors: my Nana, Augusta Emansky, and my former professor, Richard Schoenwald, for always believing in me and for teaching me to believe in myself. I know that wherever they are, they are smiling down on me.

Thanks also to all my wonderful friends without whom life would be a lonely journey. To my wonderful parents, Barbara and Ron Sickmen. To my mother for her passion and the unconditional love and support with which she nurtures me. I hope to someday be half the mother she is. To my father for passing on to me drive, ambition, and a good work ethic; I am lucky to have such a loving and supportive father. And to my in-laws, Marcia and Ernie Zied, for giving me my wonderful husband, Brian. He is my true soul mate. I thank him for his unconditional love, support, and encouragement, and for always going the extra mile to help me pursue and achieve my dreams. Thank-you to the two lights in my life, Spencer and Eli. I am beyond blessed to be the mother of two such kind, sweet, and extraordinary people who fill me with pride every day. And to Maria "Linda" Arevalo for loving my boys and helping me take care of them as I pursue a career that means so much to me.

Introduction

My mother, a very intelligent, well-read woman, is full of energy and a lust for life. She enjoys music, theater, her grandchildren, and, much to her chagrin, food. She's battled with her weight for decades and has worked hard to understand the basics of nutrition. So I was very surprised when I asked her what brand of yogurt she eats and she answered, "I stay away from yogurt because it has too much sugar."

My mother's renunciation of yogurt, a food she loves, is an example of how misinformation leads to our making less-than-optimal food decisions. Yogurt contains natural sugar and is a great source of important nutrients such as calcium, especially for a woman my mother's age.

I am a registered dietitian and a spokesperson for the American Dietetic Association. It is my goal to clarify the often conflicting information you hear every day about food and nutrition and to help you incorporate the nutritional science of the new Dietary Guidelines for Americans, as well as of the MyPyramid Food Guidance System, into your daily life. The guidelines evolved from an analysis of the latest scientific information by the Dietary Guidelines Advisory Committee (DGAC), which was appointed by the secretaries of the U.S. Department of Health and Human Services (HHS) and the U.S. Department of Agriculture (USDA). These guidelines are the foundation for the MyPyramid Food Guidance System.

In this book, you'll learn how to create your own healthful, delicious diet according to your specific needs and preferences, whether your goal is to lose weight, gain weight, have more energy, or manage or prevent diet-related health conditions.

Not only do the Dietary Guidelines and the MyPyramid Food Guidance System contain recommendations for incorporating nutritional powerhouse foods like fruits, vegetables, and whole grains into your diet, but they cite the importance of not specifically counting calories but making calories count. For the first time, the new guidelines give us some wiggle room to be more flexible in our food selections. For each calorie level, a certain number of discretionary calories is allotted. These calories are essentially the extra calories we earn once we've met our daily quotas for nutrient-rich foods in each food category. We can use these extra calories to:

- Help ourselves to larger portions of nutrient-rich foods.
- Indulge in alcoholic beverages or sweets.
- Eat foods from various food groups that already contain extra fat or sugar.
- Add butter or other solid fats to foods we're already consuming.

While not all of us can afford these extra calories (for example, if we're trying to lose weight), it's nice to know some of the low-nutrient foods we enjoy can still be part of our diet, at least sometimes; we don't have to give up *all* the foods that give us pleasure. In this book you'll learn what your estimated calorie needs are, as well as the dietary pattern you can use as a building block to create your own unique daily meal plans. You will also learn what counts as a portion for various foods in each food category and will be given tools to help you fit many of your favorite foods into your daily meal plans and overall dietary pattern.

Every year, new diet books scream the message that if we want to lose weight or improve our health, we need to:

- Avoid a particular food or food group.
- Eat only at or until specific times of the day.
- Combine certain types of foods with one another at mealtimes.
- Not eat past a certain hour.

The tremendous sales of diet books prove that many of us are constantly in search of the perfect diet—one that will help us lose our love handles or spare tires, drop a clothing size, get more toned or more muscular bodies, or simply weigh less. And while each so-called diet book may offer an idea or a strategy that can help in our quest to lose weight quickly and easily, most of these books encourage very restrictive, low-calorie diets that ask us to drastically cut back on many of the foods and food groups we enjoy, such as carbohydrates and high-fat foods.

When I use the word *diet* in this book, it's not in a restrictive sense. I'm a registered dietitian, not a food cop. You'll discover that you don't have to severely restrict calories or avoid any food group to achieve your health or nutrition goals. I love chocolate, for example; I eat it but still have a healthful, balanced diet. You, too, can include your favorite foods in your diet, and this book will teach you how. In addition, I want to help you change your mindset, just as I changed mine after years of going on and off diets. Too many of us (myself included when I was a teenager) are seduced by the idea of taking weight off fast and pay little regard to whether the diet we go on is sustainable or even healthful and well balanced over the long term. I want you to think less about going "on" or "off" any diet program and more about making a balanced, sustainable, and nutritious overall eating plan a part of your life.

This book will help you create your own healthful eating plan based on the new Dietary Guidelines for Americans and the MyPyramid Food Guidance System. You'll see that even processed or fast foods, ice cream, and butter can fit into an otherwise nutrient-packed diet. You'll be able to enjoy eating, without feeling deprived, because if you don't enjoy your food, as we all know, you'll eventually return to the habits that contributed to your becoming nutritionally challenged in the first place.

PART ONE

So What Are the Guidelines and How Can You Fit Them into Your Life?

1
Sitting Down to Dinner with Uncle Sam

We are all in search of the perfect diet, a quick and easy way to help us look and feel better. Some of us have diet-influenced conditions that we want to control or better manage, such as high blood pressure or type 2 diabetes, or maybe we just want to use the latest scientific information to fine-tune our current dietary habits. The problem is that so many diet books and commercial weight-loss programs recommend restrictive eating practices. They tell us to:

- Avoid high-carbohydrate foods, especially pasta, bread, cereal, potatoes, and sugar.
- Limit or restrict the intake of fruits and vegetables.
- Avoid red meat.
- Shun dairy foods.
- Eat only raw foods or certain-colored foods.

Of course, no one diet book asks you to eliminate all these foods (if it did, we'd have nothing left to eat!). But scores of books do recommend that we limit many foods that are known to provide vital nutrients and can be part—sometimes a big part—of a healthful, balanced, nutrient-rich diet. To illustrate this, I've put together a list of foods and beverages that many popular diet books encourage you to minimize if not avoid entirely, at least while you actively try to lose weight while following their programs.

Are These Really No-No Foods?

alcoholic beverages

bagels

balsamic vinegar

barbecue sauce

beans

beef

beets

bread

breath mints

caffeinated beverages

candy

carrots

chewing gum

coleslaw

corn

cottage cheese

cough drops

cough syrups

crackers

cream soups

doughnuts

egg yolks

farmer cheese

French dressing

fried fish and shellfish

fruit

fruit juice

gravy

hot dogs

ice cream

ketchup

milk

parsnips

pasta

peas

pork

potatoes

poultry

ready-to-eat cereals

sandwich meats

snack foods

soft drinks

stick margarine

table sugar

thousand island dressing

tuna fish salad

veal

white flour

yams

yogurt

The good news is that you won't have to give up *any* of your favorite foods to follow a diet that's consistent with the Dietary Guidelines. You may have to eat smaller portions, especially of foods that are high in fat and/or added sugar. But you'll find that you can actually consume a lot of food—perhaps more food than you currently do—because you will likely choose the nutrient-dense foods within each category more often than you do now. This will help you to take in fewer total calories but still feel satisfied. Also, because no specific food is a "no-no," and all foods that you enjoy can be worked into your overall dietary pattern, you may avoid feeling deprived the way you do on other diets.

No one diet is absolutely perfect, of course, but the new Dietary Guidelines do provide the best, most comprehensive, and most up-to-date scientific information to lay the foundation for a healthful, balanced, and sustainable eating plan. This plan does not discriminate against any one food or food group but instead encourages you to choose nutrient-rich foods and beverages that will help you manage your weight, control or prevent diet-related ailments, and fill any nutrient gaps in your diet. So whether your goal is to shed weight, gain weight, lower your blood pressure or blood cholesterol levels, manage your diabetes, prevent diseases like heart disease and cancer, or simply have a well-balanced, nutrient-rich, and satisfying diet, the science-based Dietary Guidelines are the perfect place to start.

What Are the Dietary Guidelines?

The guidelines, published jointly by the U.S. Department of Health and Human Services (HHS) and the U.S. Department of Agriculture (USDA) every five years, are designed to promote optimal nutrition, prevent disease, and serve as the foundation for nutrition policies. The recommendations are based on a preponderance of scientific evidence about which dietary practices will lower the risk of chronic disease and promote health. And while you can certainly benefit by following even a few of the guidelines (for example, eating more fruits and vegetables than you do now), all the recommendations in the new guidelines, taken as a whole, will provide a roadmap by which you can steer your own unique course toward more healthful and balanced, yet still enjoyable, eating.

The deliberately simplistic MyPyramid graphic on page 10 will remind you to choose healthful foods and to and make physical activity a part of your day, every day. MyPyramid encourages you to look for the following in your food choices:

- *Variety*: Eat foods within all the food groups (fruits, vegetables, grains, meat and beans, and milk) and subgroups (for example, dark green, deep-orange, and starchy vegetables).
- *Proportionality*: Eat more fruits, vegetables, whole grains, and fat-free or low-fat milk products; eat fewer foods that are high in saturated or trans fats, added sugars, cholesterol, salt, and alcohol.
- *Moderation*: Choose foods that are prepared in a way that makes them lower in saturated and trans fats, added sugars, cholesterol, salt, and alcohol.
- *Activity*: Incorporate more moderate or vigorous daily physical activity into your schedule.

MyPyramid

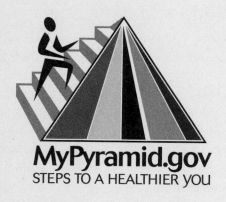

MyPyramid.gov
STEPS TO A HEALTHIER YOU

Source: U.S. Department of Agriculture

The Dietary Guidelines emphasize foods and beverages as the most important sources of nutrients and healthful compounds. Of course, not everyone will be able to meet his or her nutritional needs through foods alone, so, in some cases, fortified foods and dietary supplements can be helpful. This book will highlight a wide range of foods and beverages that you can choose from all the major food categories, day to day. If you are pregnant, have a medical condition, or follow a vegetarian or otherwise restricted diet and feel that you cannot meet your nutritional needs with foods or beverages alone, see your physician and a registered dietitian to discuss dietary supplements.

The Dietary Guidelines are ideals, and you may initially find them challenging to follow. My goal is to help you adapt the guidelines to your individual needs and to come closer to achieving the ideals on your own terms. This doesn't mean that you have to follow the guidelines precisely and perfectly, but you can use them as a starting point to improve your intake of key foods (for example, fruits, vegetables, and whole grains) and the nutrients they contain. So even if you find it tough to get all the recommended foods into your diet—and when I say *diet*, I don't mean this in the restrictive sense, but in the pattern of what you eat—the guidelines can help you create a well-rounded dietary plan that you can easily follow, not for a short time but for life!

Changes to the Dietary Guidelines

The current Dietary Guidelines differ in scope and purpose from past versions because they are oriented toward policymakers, health-care providers, registered dietitians, and other nutrition educators, rather than toward the general public, as were previous versions. They also contain more technical information. But don't despair. In this book, I'll help you create your own personal dietary and physical activity plans based on the new guidelines. Before you get started, though, here's a sample of a diet that is consistent with the Dietary Guidelines:

- *Menus for you*: Throughout most of this book and in the sample two-week meal plans (see chapter 7), I use 2,000 calories as a reference level to be consistent with the Nutrition Facts panels on food labels. Your individual calorie needs, as well as your corresponding meal plan, may differ depending on your age, weight, height, gender, and activity level (see chapter 2 and appendix B to determine your individual calorie needs). Once you determine your estimated calorie needs, see chapter 7 to find the corresponding daily meal plan.

- *Personal palate pleasers*: The recommendations in the Dietary Guidelines are for Americans older than two years of age.

What's great about these new guidelines is that they allow you to choose a wide range of foods and beverages. Whether you're a vegan, you eat a lot of ethnic foods because of your heritage or individual food preferences, or you don't drink milk because you're allergic or don't like the taste, you'll be given the tools to adapt the guidelines to help you maximize your nutrient intake. For example, if you are a vegetarian or a vegan and you don't eat meat of any kind, you can choose from a variety of other foods, such as beans, nuts, and seeds, to get protein and other key nutrients (see chapter 3 and appendix A to find meat alternatives).

- *The right calories*: The new Dietary Guidelines clearly emphasize balancing calorie intake with expenditure, which is crucial for long-term weight management and to prevent weight gain as you grow older. In the wake of the low-carbohydrate craze (and before that, the low-fat phase), it's great that the emphasis is back where it should be—on calories. And while the Dietary Guidelines do say that calories count, *they do not ask you to count calories*. Neither will I. If you, like many of my clients, choose to count calories, however, I've provided you with calorie counts for all of the recipes, as well as calorie estimates for foods in different food categories (see the food lists in chapter 3). If you are trying to lose weight or prevent weight gain or regain, it's important to keep an eye on calories, especially with foods that provide extra calories but few, if any, nutrients. These include solid fats like butter, foods made with solid fats or trans fats, fried foods, sugar that's found in cola or candy or added to foods, and alcoholic beverages, to name a few. The information and the resources in this book will arm you with tools to help you reduce your calorie intake if you want to or need to.

- *Better ways to move*: The new guidelines encourage a lot of daily activity—a whopping 30 to 90 minutes a day, more than ever before. For the first time, the guidelines distinguish between the amount of exercise and physical activity that is required to stay healthy and the amount that is necessary to prevent weight gain as we age, as well as weight regain in people who have previously lost weight. You'll learn how much and what types of daily physical activity are right for you. You'll also discover fresh ways to easily and painlessly incorporate new movements into your day to keep yourself strong and fit and manage your weight. You will learn how to make physical activity a permanent part of your life (see chapter 4).

- *A colorful life*: The new Dietary Guidelines recommend a daily minimum of 4½ cups of fruits and vegetables. The guidelines also specify recommended weekly intakes of different colors and subcategories of vegetables, such as dark green vegetables like broccoli and kale, deep-orange vegetables like carrots and sweet potatoes, starchy vegetables like corn and white potatoes, and legumes like peas and lentils. Eating fruits and vegetables is enormously beneficial because of the nutrients, the fiber, and the antioxidants they contain. Consuming a diet that's rich in fruits and vegetables may help you prevent stroke, type 2 diabetes, some types of cancer, and other ailments. It may also help you manage your weight (see chapter 4).

- *The whole grain of truth*: For the first time, the guidelines encourage you to consume at least half of your total grains from whole grains. For someone who consumes 2,000 calories a day, that's six 1-ounce equivalents of grains a day, with at least half of those from whole grains. Research suggests that diets that contain a lot of whole grains can reduce the risk for heart disease and type 2 diabetes.

- *Desirable dairy*: The new guidelines now place dairy foods alongside fruits, vegetables, and whole grains as "foods to encourage." For the first time, they specify the equivalent of three cups of milk a day for people who consume at least 1,600 calories a day. In addition to milk, both yogurt and cheese can be counted toward your daily recommended amounts. Of course, not everyone drinks milk or consumes enough dairy foods to meet his or her nutrient needs, so the guidelines provide recommendations for other foods that will help make up for certain missing nutrients like calcium. These foods include legumes, fish, tofu made with calcium, dark green leafy vegetables, and calcium-fortified orange juice (see chapter 3 for a complete list of nondairy calcium-rich foods).

• *An oil change*: The new Dietary Guidelines encourage a daily equivalent of 27 grams or 6 teaspoons of oil—that includes vegetable oils and soft trans fat–free margarines that are found in processed foods or added during cooking or at the table. These oils are rich in polyunsaturated fatty acids (as well as in essential fatty acids that we must obtain through food sources), which are necessary for metabolism. They also contain vitamin E, a fat-soluble antioxidant that retards fat rancidity in foods. The new Dietary Guidelines bump up their fat recommendation; previously, it was 20 to 30 percent of your diet. Now, it is 20 to 35 percent, and they encourage you to get any additional fat, if you choose to, from unsaturated sources and to limit saturated and trans fats to no more than 10 percent of your total daily calories.

• *A spoonful of sugar*: Although the new guidelines don't set a specific cap on sugar, if you consume foods in the proportions recommended for your particular calorie level, it's tough to take in too much sugar. Nevertheless, it's a good idea to try to limit portions, especially when you consume sugary foods such as candy, nondiet soda, juices that aren't 100 percent fruit juice, cakes, cookies, jams, and jellies, to name a few. The Dietary Reference Intake Reports of the National Academy of Sciences Food and Nutrition Board currently suggests that not more than 25 percent of your total calories should come from added sugars. Although this far exceeds the World Health Organization's upper limit of 10 percent of total calories from sugar each day, following a dietary pattern consistent with the Dietary Guidelines will help you achieve optimal health and will inevitably limit your consumption of sugar and other low-nutrient foods.

• *A smaller shaker of salt*: The guidelines note that nearly all Americans consume substantially more salt than they need and that decreasing salt intake is advisable to reduce the risk of high blood pressure. The recommendation is to consume less than 2,300 mg (approximately 1 teaspoon of salt) per day. On average, the meal plans in this book (see chapter 7) provide less than 2,300 mg of sodium a day. The recommendation for people who may be salt-sensitive—those with hypertension, or those who are black or middle aged or older—is no more than 1,500 mg a day. See chapter 5 for tips to help you identify lower-sodium foods and to find tasty salt substitutions you can use when you cook.

* *Pumped up with potassium*: The guidelines recommend consuming a diet that's rich in potassium, a mineral that blunts the effect of salt on blood pressure and may also reduce the risk of developing kidney stones and possibly bone loss as we get older. The recommended intake of potassium for adolescents and adults is 4,700 mg/day. The recommended intake for children 1 to 3 years of age is 3,000 mg/day; 4 to 8 years, 3,800 mg/day; and 9 to 13 years, 4,500 mg/day. Leafy green vegetables, fruit from vines, and root vegetables are great sources of potassium. And while meat, milk, and cereal products also contain potassium, it is not in the form that's most absorbable by the body. The following table contains a list of potassium-rich foods and beverages:

Food, Standard Amount*	Potassium (in milligrams)
Sweet potato, baked, 1 potato	694
Tomato paste, ¼ cup	664
Beet greens, cooked, ½ cup	655
Potato, baked, flesh, 1 potato	610
White beans, canned, ½ cup	595
Yogurt, plain, nonfat, 8 oz.	579
Tomato puree, ½ cup	549
Clams, canned, 3 oz.	534
Yogurt, plain, lowfat, 8 oz.	531
Prune juice, ¾ cup	530
Carrot juice, ¾ cup	517
Blackstrap molasses, 1 tbsp.	498

Food, Standard Amount*	Potassium (in milligrams)
Halibut, cooked, 3 oz.	490
Soybeans, green, cooked, ½ cup	485
Tuna, yellowfin, cooked, 3 oz.	484
Lima beans, cooked, ½ cup	478
Winter squash, cooked, ½ cup	448
Soybeans, mature, cooked, ½ cup	443
Rockfish, Pacific, cooked, 3 oz.	442
Cod, Pacific, cooked, 3 oz.	439
Bananas, 1 medium	422
Spinach, cooked, ½ cup	419
Tomato juice, ¾ cup	417
Tomato sauce, ½ cup	405
Peaches, dried, uncooked, ¼ cup	398
Prunes, stewed, ½ cup	398
Milk, nonfat, 1 cup	382
Pork chop, center loin, cooked, 3 oz.	382
Apricots, dried, uncooked, ¼ cup	378
Rainbow trout, cooked, 3 oz.	375
Pork loin, center rib (roasts), lean, roasted, 3 oz.	371
Buttermilk, cultured, low-fat, 1 cup	370
Cantaloupe, ¼ medium	368
1% milk, 1 cup	366
2% milk, 1 cup	366
Honeydew melon, ⅛ medium	365
Lentils, cooked, ½ cup	365
Plantains, cooked, ½ cup	358
Kidney beans, cooked, ½ cup	357
Orange juice, ¾ cup	355
Split peas, cooked, ½ cup	355
Yogurt, plain, whole milk, 8 oz.	352

Source: ARS Nutrient Database for Standard Reference, Release 16-1.
*These standard amounts may be more or less than the amount you actually consume.

- *Sweet pleasures*: For the first time, the Dietary Guidelines provide you with extra calories that you can use for any food or beverage your heart desires—but there is a catch. To earn those extra calories, you are expected to consume the most nutrient-dense foods that exist within each food category. This means nonfat or low-fat milk, yogurt, and cheese; lean meats like white meat chicken without the skin and sirloin; and fruits, vegetables, and grains made without any extra added sugar or fat. Once you consume foods from each food category in the allotted amounts, you can then use some or all of your discretionary calories as you see fit—for a 2,000-calorie diet, that's 267 calories. You can spend them on any foods or beverages you desire, even if they're fried and greasy, sugary, or alcoholic. Or, alternatively, you can just help yourself to a larger portion of some of the foods you're already eating, like steak or salad dressing. Knowing that you can have a satisfying helping of a food you love or can indulge in any food or beverage you love minus the guilt is a great incentive to fill up on nutrient-dense foods most of the time. If you're trying to lose weight, you may want to forgo at least some of these extra calories or use just a portion of them. That, coupled with extra physical activity or exercise, can help you to create a calorie deficit and will promote weight loss.

- *Some wine*: The Dietary Guidelines recognize that for certain people, consuming some alcohol may provide health benefits. For example, in middle-aged and older adults, one or two alcoholic beverages a day is associated with a reduced risk of death from all causes, as well as a reduced risk for coronary heart disease. The guidelines also recognize that despite these potential benefits for some populations, alcohol may have negative effects, depending on how much is consumed and the age and other characteristics of the person who consumes it. Because alcohol has few essential nutrients, the calories from alcohol are counted as discretionary calories (see chapter 3 for calories in alcohol). For people who wish to drink, if alcohol consumption is not contraindicated, the recommendation is up to one drink a day for women and up to two drinks a day for

When You Should *Not* Drink

- If you cannot restrict your alcohol intake
- If you may become pregnant
- If you are pregnant or nursing
- If you are a child or an adolescent
- If you have certain specific medical conditions, such as an ulcer or liver disease
- If you are taking prescription or over-the-counter medications that alcohol can interfere with
- If you plan to drive or operate machinery or perform any activities that require attention, skill, or coordination

men. One drink is defined as 12 ounces of beer, 5 ounces of wine, or 1½ ounces of 80-proof distilled spirits.

- *Keep food safe*: The guidelines emphasize the need to keep food safe to eat. That's something many of us often neglect or don't think twice about. Remember when you ordered a deli sandwich and the man who prepared it didn't wear gloves? Or how about the last time you left a fresh roasted chicken in your car for two hours when it was 90 degrees Fahrenheit outside (one of my good friends did that!)? Or how about the butcher who handled raw meat, put it in plastic wrap, and gave it to you to put next to the other items in your grocery cart?

   There are countless situations in which we don't think about food safety, but keeping foods safe for consumption is key. The following tips based on the Dietary Guidelines can help you keep food safe and avoid microbial foodborne illness:

   - Clean hands, food-contact surfaces, and raw foods like fruits and vegetables.
   - Do *not* wash or rinse meat or poultry.
   - Separate raw, cooked, and ready-to-eat foods while shopping for, preparing, or storing foods.
   - Cook foods to a safe temperature to kill microorganisms.
   - Refrigerate perishable foods promptly and defrost foods properly.

- Avoid raw (unpasteurized) milk or any products made from unpasteurized milk.
- Avoid raw or partially cooked eggs or foods containing raw eggs, raw or undercooked meat and poultry, unpasteurized juices, and raw sprouts.
- Check expiration dates on the perishables you buy.
- When in doubt about a food, throw it out.

For more food safety information, see "Resources" at the back of this book.

Using the Guidelines

As you read this book, you'll see that the new Dietary Guidelines provide a wonderful starting point for you to create your own nutritious eating plan and overall healthful lifestyle. Turning the recommendations into real-world, sustainable practices is admittedly no easy task, however.

This book will make tangible the principles and ideas of the new Dietary Guidelines for Americans and the MyPyramid Food Guidance System. I'll show you how to create your own unique plan of action that details what to do, how to do it, and how you'll benefit from it. Thus you will be guided and inspired to follow not the fad of the moment but the facts, based on the latest science, about what makes up a healthful and balanced nutrient-rich diet.

2
How to Make the Guidelines Your Own in 7 Steps

Now that you've been introduced to the new Dietary Guidelines and MyPyramid, are you ready, willing, and able to make some positive behavioral changes in your dietary and physical activity habits? Taking action is not the problem—you've undoubtedly done that plenty of times. The real problem is that you might start to make changes only to stop your efforts altogether at a later point. Remember when you cut back on carbs, curtailed your wine intake, or stopped eating dessert? Maybe you joined a gym. You have no problem changing your behaviors, but sustaining them—learning to make them part of your life—is the hard part. You may be asking yourself, right this minute, whether it's even worth the effort to tackle some of your nutritional or fitness challenges, especially if all of your efforts will only be short-lived.

I hope that after you read this book, you'll become conscious of the habits that prevent you from achieving your diet and health goals, whether you desire to eat more nutritious foods, be in better shape, lower your cholesterol, or lose or gain a few pounds.

I think you'll discover that making even a *few* small changes in your life can have a big impact on your overall health, body weight, energy level, and feelings of wellness. You may even realize that certain changes that you thought would be too difficult are far easier than you expected. I'm here to guide and motivate you toward making realistic changes. I'll help you learn to eat nutritiously and to exercise according to the principles encouraged by the Dietary Guidelines and MyPyramid. So let's begin our journey; we're in this together.

Eating the Guidelines Way

All I ask is that you commit eighteen days—just a blip of time in the context of your life—so that we can create an eating plan based on your unique nutrient and calorie needs, lifestyle, food preferences, and, let's not forget, budget. During these eighteen days, you will take the following seven steps toward improving your food and nutrient intake. To get started, read through each of the seven steps. Then I'll show you how I followed the same steps in pursuit of a better, more balanced diet.

- **Step 1: Keep track.** For three days (preferably on two week-days and one weekend day), keep track of all the foods, beverages, breath mints, and sticks of chewing gum that pass your lips, using the Daily Food and Fitness Tracker on page 22. First, complete the first two columns of the tracker, "Food or Beverage" and "Amount Consumed." Keeping tabs on what and how much you eat for a few days will likely be an eye-opening exercise. You'll learn to identify your food habits and objectively assess how balanced your overall diet is. This will be especially helpful if you are an automatic eater and often choose foods or beverages without really thinking about them because that's what you've always done.

- **Step 2: Get familiar with the food groups.** Use the food lists in chapter 3 and appendix A to determine how many portions of foods and beverages from the various food categories you've consumed—fruits, vegetables, grains, meat and beans, oils, and discretionary calories—on each of the three days. You can check off items and add up totals using your Daily Food and Fitness Tracker.

- **Step 3: Determine your estimated calorie needs.** Use the chart on page 24 to figure out how many calories you need to

Daily Food and Fitness Tracker

Food or Beverage	Amount Consumed	Fruits	Vegetables	Whole Grains	Other Grains	Meat and Beans	Milk	Oils	Discretionary Calories
Breakfast									
Lunch									
Dinner									
Snacks/desserts									
Totals for the day									
Dietary Guidelines goals for the day									
Total daily physical activity	Circle a 1 for each 10-minute interval completed 1 1 1 1 1 1 1 1 1								

22

maintain your current body weight, based on your gender, age, and activity level. Keep in mind that this is just an estimate and that your individual calorie needs may vary (you'll need to keep an eye on your body weight and make appropriate adjustments if this calorie level seems too high or too low).

Calorie levels are provided for each year of childhood, from two to eighteen years, and for adults in five-year increments. Calorie levels are based on the estimated energy requirements (EER) and the activity levels from the *Institute of Medicine Dietary Reference Intakes Macronutrients Report*, 2002.

Again, the chart provides a general estimate of how many calories you can consume to maintain your body weight. If you want to do the math yourself and use formulas that registered dietitians and other health professionals use to take into account your weight and height as well, see appendix B.

If your goal is to lose or gain weight, go to step 4. If your goal is to maintain your weight, go to step 5.

- **Step 4: Adjust your calorie level if you want to lose or gain weight.** If you want to lose weight, find the food plan associated with a lower calorie level to create a daily calorie deficit and promote weight loss. For example, if your calorie needs are 2,400 a day, you can cut back to 2,000. If you also do an additional 30 minutes of daily exercise, you'll be on course to lose about 1 pound each week. If your goal is to gain weight, you can easily add calories by consuming larger portions of energy-dense foods such as nuts, nut butters, and vegetable oils.

- **Step 5: Match your calorie level with the appropriate food plan.** Use the table on page 25 to determine how much to consume from each food category daily. Fill in the "Dietary Guidelines goals for the day" on your Daily Food and Fitness Tracker.

- **Step 6: Compare your actual intake with the Dietary Guidelines goals for the day.** Use the food lists in chapter 3 to determine how many portions of foods and beverages you consumed from each category, and check these off on your Daily Food and Fitness Tracker. See how your actual intake

MyPyramid Food Intake Pattern Calorie Levels

	MALES			FEMALES		
	Activity Level			Activity Level		
Age	Sedentary[a]	Moderately Active[b]	Active[c]	Sedentary[a]	Moderately Active[b]	Active[c]
2	1,000	1,000	1,000	1,000	1,000	1,000
3	1,000	1,400	1,400	1,000	1,200	1,400
4	1,200	1,400	1,600	1,200	1,400	1,400
5	1,200	1,400	1,600	1,200	1,400	1,600
6	1,400	1,600	1,800	1,200	1,400	1,600
7	1,400	1,600	1,800	1,200	1,600	1,800
8	1,400	1,600	2,000	1,400	1,600	1,800
9	1,600	1,800	2,000	1,400	1,600	1,800
10	1,600	1,800	2,200	1,400	1,800	2,000
11	1,800	2,000	2,200	1,600	1,800	2,000
12	1,800	2,200	2,400	1,600	2,000	2,200
13	2,000	2,200	2,600	1,600	2,000	2,200
14	2,000	2,400	2,800	1,800	2,000	2,400
15	2,200	2,600	3,000	1,800	2,000	2,400
16	2,400	2,800	3,200	1,800	2,000	2,400
17	2,400	2,800	3,200	1,800	2,000	2,400
18	2,400	2,800	3,200	1,800	2,000	2,400
19–20	2,600	2,800	3,000	2,000	2,200	2,400
21–25	2,400	2,800	3,000	2,000	2,200	2,400
26–30	2,400	2,600	3,000	1,800	2,000	2,400
31–35	2,400	2,600	3,000	1,800	2,000	2,200
36–40	2,400	2,600	2,800	1,800	2,000	2,200
41–45	2,200	2,600	2,800	1,800	2,000	2,200
46–50	2,200	2,400	2,800	1,800	2,000	2,200
51–55	2,200	2,400	2,800	1,600	1,800	2,200
56–60	2,200	2,400	2,600	1,600	1,800	2,200
61–65	2,000	2,400	2,600	1,600	1,800	2,000
66–70	2,000	2,200	2,600	1,600	1,800	2,000
71–75	2,000	2,200	2,600	1,600	1,800	2,000
76+	2,000	2,000	2,400	1,600	1,800	2,000

Source: USDA's mypyramid.gov.

Sedentary = less than 30 minutes a day of moderate physical activity in addition to daily activities.

[b]Moderately Active = at least 30 minutes up to 60 minutes a day of moderate physical activity in addition to daily activities.

[c]Active = 60 or more minutes a day of moderate physical activity in addition to daily activities.

Suggested Daily Amount of Food from Each Food Group											
CALORIE LEVEL											
Food Group	1,000	1,200	1,400	1,600	1,800	2,000	2,200	2,400	2,600	2,800	3,000	3,200
Fruits (cups)	1	1	1.5	1.5	1.5	2	2	2	2	2.5	2.5	2.5
Vegetables (cups)	1	1.5	1.5	2	2.5	2.5	3	3	3.5	3.5	4	4
Whole grains (1 oz. equivalents)	1.5	2	2.5	3	3	3	3.5	4	4.5	5	5	5
Other grains (1 oz. equivalents)	1.5	2	2.5	2	3	3	3.5	4	4.5	5	5	5
Meat and beans (1 oz. equivalents)	2	3	4	5	5	5.5	6	6.5	6.5	7	7	7
Milk (cups)	2	2	2	3	3	3	3	3	3	3	3	3
Oils (grams)	15	17	17	22	24	27	29	31	34	36	44	51
Discretionary calories	165	171	171	132	195	267	290	362	410	426	512	648

Source: U.S. Department of Agriculture

compares with your Dietary Guidelines goals. Did you go way over in any food groups? Did you miss any other food groups entirely? Can you identify a pattern, and are there particular areas where you need improvement? Use what you learn from this exercise to set food-related goals for yourself.

- **Step 7: Eat the Dietary Guidelines way for two weeks.** Try to incorporate as many of the food recommendations into your diet as you can. You can either follow the two weeks of daily menu plans (see chapter 7), plan your own meals using the menus as templates, or do a combination of the two. If you choose to create your own personal menus, be sure to use the Daily Food and Fitness Tracker to record your food and beverage intake during the two weeks, as well as the food lists in chapter 3 and in appendix A. This exercise will help you become familiar with each of the food categories, as well as with the many choices you have within each category.

Tips for Building More Nutritious and Delicious Meals

Following are some tips to help you turn the recommendations for eating fruits, vegetables, lean meats and beans, and milk into daily and weekly habits.

Fruit

At breakfast, you can

- Top cereal with sliced bananas, strawberries, or peaches.
- Add bananas or applesauce to pancake batter.
- Add fresh blueberries, raspberries, or strawberries on top of plain pancakes or waffles.
- Mix fresh berries, crushed pineapple, or dried fruit with low-fat or fat-free yogurt.
- Fill half a cantaloupe with low-fat yogurt or cottage cheese.

At lunch, you can

- Round out a sandwich with a banana, an apple, an orange, or fresh fruit salad from a salad bar.
- Top salads with slices of a Granny Smith apple, grapes, oranges, or raisins or other dried fruit.
- Add apple or banana slices to peanut butter sandwiches.

At dinner, you can

- Garnish your meals with fresh fruit slices.
- Serve grapefruit sections with vinaigrette as an appetizer.
- Make a salsa with fruit to top fish or chicken.
- Add fruit such as pineapple or peaches to kabobs as part of a barbecue meal.

At snack or dessert time, you can

- Pack grapes or blueberries in a baggie or carry a small container of natural applesauce with you.
- Keep small boxes of raisins, dried cherries, or other dried fruits (prunes, apricots, cranberries) in your backpack or desk drawer.
- Keep a fresh fruit bowl with apples, oranges, clementines, bananas, and pears on your desk or kitchen counter and restock it every few days.
- Have a baked apple with cinnamon, fresh fruit, a fruit smoothie made with low-fat or nonfat yogurt, or a fresh fruit salad.

- Top frozen yogurt with berries or slices of kiwi fruit.
- Have a frozen juice bar (made with 100 percent fruit juice).
- Have some frozen grapes or bananas.
- Dip fresh fruit slices such as strawberries or melon chunks into low-fat yogurt or low-fat vanilla pudding.

Vegetables

- Use a microwave to quickly zap vegetables; white or sweet potatoes can be cooked quickly this way.
- Vary your veggie choices to keep meals interesting.
- Try crunchy vegetables, raw or lightly steamed.

At breakfast, you can

- Add onions and red and green peppers to dishes made with eggs or egg whites (see the recipes in chapter 8).
- Add canned tomatoes or a fresh cut-up tomato to a toasted pita or an English muffin and top with shredded mozzarella cheese for a breakfast pizza.
- Make sweet potato pancakes (see the recipe in chapter 8).

At lunch, you can

- Have vegetable soup or a side salad with half a sandwich.
- Make a sandwich with grilled vegetables such as eggplant, red or green peppers, and zucchini.
- Have a large colorful salad with a mix of crunchy vegetables, beans, or nuts.

At dinner, you can

- Nosh on raw vegetables (like baby carrots or cherry tomatoes) while you make dinner.
- Have vegetable soup as a starter.
- Make a vegetable-heavy stir-fry.
- Have salad as a main course, with grilled fish or slices of steak or chicken.

- Make a baked sweet potato or sweet potato French fries (see the recipe in chapter 8).
- Layer a lasagna with grilled vegetables.
- Add shredded carrots, cut-up fresh or canned tomatoes, or chopped zucchini when you make baked ziti, meatloaf, or a casserole.
- Top a lightly sautéed vegetable medley with pasta (instead of the other way around).
- Make or order a pizza loaded with vegetables (mushrooms, green peppers, and onions).
- Use pureed, cooked vegetables such as potatoes to thicken stews, soups, and gravies (these add flavor, nutrients, and texture).
- Grill vegetables at your next barbecue; corn, eggplant, zucchini, and carrots can be grilled alone or as part of a kebob with some lean meat or fish.

At snack or dessert time, you can

- Have cut-up fresh vegetables—broccoli, red and green peppers, celery sticks, carrots, or cauliflower—with a low-fat yogurt dip (made with low-sodium onion broth mix) or low-fat salad dressing.
- Add shredded carrots or zucchini when you make whole-grain muffins.

Grains
Here are some tips to boost your intake of whole grains (we already eat enough refined ones!).
At breakfast, you can

- Have whole-grain cereal with low-fat or nonfat milk and fresh fruit.
- Top low-fat or nonfat yogurt with a crunchy whole-grain cereal, and round that out with fresh fruit or orange juice.
- Top a toasted whole-wheat or other whole-grain bread, English muffin, or pita with egg or egg whites, low-fat cheese, or trans fat–free margarine.

- Mix ½ cup of a high-fiber, whole-grain cereal with ½ cup of your usual cereal, if you normally don't eat whole-grain cereal.
- Add wheat germ to low-fat or nonfat yogurt.
- Substitute whole-wheat or oat flour for up to half the flour (the recipe may need a little more leavening) when you make pancakes, waffles, muffins, or other flour-based products.

At lunch, you can

- Use whole-grain breads to make sandwiches.
- Make a whole-wheat pasta salad with vegetables and beans.
- Have a cup of barley soup.

At dinner, you can

- Have brown rice or whole-wheat pasta.
- Use brown rice to stuff cabbage, baked red or green peppers, or tomatoes.
- Use whole-wheat macaroni to make macaroni and cheese.
- Add whole grains in mixed dishes, such as barley in vegetable soup or stews and bulgur wheat in casseroles or stir-fries.
- Create a whole-grain pilaf with a mixture of barley, wild rice, brown rice, broth, and spices.
- Try using an unsweetened, whole-grain, ready-to-eat cereal as croutons in a salad or in place of crackers with soup.
- Use whole-grain bread or cracker crumbs in a meatloaf.
- Use rolled oats or a crushed, unsweetened whole-grain cereal as breading for baked chicken, fish, veal cutlets, or eggplant parmesan.
- Freeze leftover cooked brown rice, bulgur, or barley; heat and serve it later as a quick side dish.

At snack or dessert time, you can

- Top whole-grain crackers with peanut butter and raisins.
- Munch on air-popped or canola oil–popped popcorn.

Meat and Beans

At breakfast, you can

- Sprinkle nuts or seeds on cereal or low-fat yogurt.
- Use egg whites to make scrambled eggs and omelets.
- Spread peanut butter on toasted whole-wheat bread.

At lunch, you can

- Have a bean-based soup as the main course.
- Add beans and legumes, such as garbanzo or kidney beans, to salads.
- Have a veggie burger or a garden burger.
- Add walnuts, pecans, or sunflower seeds to salads instead of, or to complement, cheese or meat.

At dinner, you can

- Choose fish more often as a main dish.
- Make chili with kidney or pinto beans.
- Make bean burritos with lentils or make enchiladas with black beans.
- Make a tofu stir-fry (see the recipe in chapter 8).
- Have bean-based soups like split pea, lentil, minestrone, or white bean.
- Have baked beans as a side dish to chicken or beef.
- Make brown rice and beans.
- Add toasted pine nuts to vegetable side dishes such as green beans or spinach.
- Top a vegetable stir-fry with toasted peanuts or cashews (instead of, or to complement, chicken or beef).

At snack or dessert time, you can

- Sprinkle nuts on low-fat frozen yogurt or low-fat ice cream.
- Make trail mix with nuts and seeds, whole-grain cereal, and dried fruit.
- Add nuts to muffin and cookie recipes.

- Put hummus (chickpeas) on pita bread or whole-grain crackers.

Milk

To incorporate more low-fat or nonfat milk, yogurt, or low-fat cheese into your diet, you can

- Drink low-fat or nonfat milk.
- Add low-fat or nonfat milk to whole-grain cereal.
- Mix whole-grain cereal with yogurt.
- Use low-fat or nonfat milk to make pancakes, waffles, and oatmeal and other hot cereals.
- Use low-fat or nonfat yogurt to make muffins.
- If you usually drink whole milk, switch gradually to fat-free milk to lower your saturated fat and calorie intake; first try reduced-fat (2%), then low-fat (1%), and finally fat-free (skim) milk.
- If you drink cappuccinos or lattes, ask for them to be made with low-fat or nonfat milk.
- Use fat-free or low-fat milk when making condensed cream soups (such as cream of tomato).
- Have fat-free or low-fat yogurt as a snack.
- Make a dip for fruits or vegetables from low-fat or nonfat yogurt and low-sodium onion broth.
- Make fruit-yogurt smoothies in the blender.
- For dessert, make chocolate or butterscotch pudding with fat-free or low-fat milk.
- Top cut-up fruit with flavored yogurt for a quick dessert.
- Top casseroles, soups, stews, or vegetables with shredded low-fat cheese.
- Add fat-free or low-fat yogurt to a baked potato.

If you avoid milk because of lactose intolerance, the most reliable way to get the nutrients in milk is to choose lactose-free alternatives within the milk group, such as cheese, yogurt, or lactose-free milk, or to consume the enzyme lactase before consuming milk products.

Calcium choices for people who don't consume milk products include calcium-fortified juices, cereals, breads, soy beverages, or rice beverages; canned fish (sardines, salmon with bones); soybeans and other soy products (soy-based beverages, soy yogurt, tempeh); certain other dried beans; and some leafy greens (collard and turnip greens, kale, bok choy). The amount of calcium that can be absorbed from these foods varies (see chpater 3 for nondairy food sources of calcium).

So there you have it—seven steps to help you make the Dietary Guidelines your own. As I said before, we're in this together.

How I Made the Guidelines My Own

I'll now share my own experiences in trying to follow the Dietary Guidelines. Even though I'm a registered dietitian and I have a relatively healthful diet, I sometimes fall into eating ruts and less-than-healthful habits, and I don't always eat as much of the good stuff—wholesome fruits and vegetables, for example—as I'd like to. So I decided that before I could teach you, I needed to make a real effort to follow the Dietary Guidelines myself. Here's how I made the Dietary Guidelines my own.

For step 1, I kept detailed food records for three days, just as you will. I won't bore you with the details for all three days but will instead describe a typical eating day. My breakfast was low-fat waffles topped with light syrup and a vegetable oil spread, and a cup of orange juice. Packaged waffles are quick and easy to pop into the toaster oven during the morning rush with my two sons. After I dropped my kids off at school, I hit the gym and in 30 minutes I walked 2 miles on the treadmill. I also did about 10 minutes of arm exercises with 3-pound free weights. That's my typical workout—quick and simple. For lunch at work, I ordered in a tuna salad sandwich on a grainy roll with American cheese, a little Russian salad dressing, lettuce, and tomato. I really love salad dressing and cheese, but to save calories (and because I get full anyway) I always opt for only half the sandwich with all the fixings, instead of having a whole sandwich minus the salad dressing and cheese. In between lunch and dinner, I raided my candy dish—that's right, I have a candy dish on my desk. It's usually filled with Hershey Kisses. I keep them there to fulfill my need for something sweet after lunch, though I admit that I nibble, almost mindlessly, on a few of these—but just a few—each day. Milk chocolate is definitely one of my vices. On this particular day, I had a few unsalted raw walnuts as well. (I also keep these on hand at work for when my stomach starts to growl midday.) Plus, I drank my once-daily can of diet Sunkist orange soda. For dinner at home with the boys, I made one of my favorite dishes—cubed eggplant and cut-up cherry tomatoes sautéed lightly in olive oil over thin spaghetti, topped with a generous sprinkling of grated parmesan cheese. My younger son, Eli, has also adopted the grated cheese habit and even dips his bean and cheese burrito into it on occasion! I drank some water with dinner and ended my eating day with an Oreo cookie and a cup of skim milk. Before bed I had more water, as I always do.

When I filled out the Daily Food and Fitness Tracker during the day, I simply recorded every food or beverage I consumed right after each meal or eating occasion (see page 34). As you can see, I tried as best I could to break down each entry—like the tuna salad sandwich—into all of its parts (for example, tuna, whole-wheat roll, American cheese, tomato, lettuce, and Russian dressing). That made it easy for me to follow step 2 and check off the appropriate food category and portion size for each food or beverage I consumed and to add up my daily totals. Of course, I realize that it's not always easy to figure out exactly what you're eating and how much of it, especially when you're eating out or not cooking the food yourself (see appendix A to learn how to record mixed meals).

For step 3, I figured out my estimated daily calorie needs. I am thirty-six years old, 5 foot 2 inches, and weigh between 115 and 117 pounds (so, let's say 116). I have lost and kept off more than 30 pounds since I was at my peak of 145 pounds in high school. I have maintained my current weight for more than seven years. Before that, I had successfully kept off 20 pounds for six years before losing the final 10. I'm sharing all of this information with you because even though I wouldn't mind losing an additional pound or two, I'm very proud of my weight loss and maintenance. My goal in following the Dietary Guidelines and eating in a

My Daily Food and Fitness Tracker

Food or Beverage	Amount Consumed	Fruits	Vegetables	Whole Grains	Other Grains	Meat and Beans	Milk	Oils	Discretionary Calories
Breakfast									
Low-fat waffles	2				2				
I Can't Believe It's Not Butter, light	1 tablespoon							1	
Light maple syrup	1 tablespoon								50
Orange juice	1 cup	1							
Lunch									
Tuna, chunk white	3 ounces					3			
Whole-wheat roll	½ (1 ounce)			1					
American cheese	1 slice						½		
Tomato	2 slices		¼						
Romaine lettuce	1 slice		⅛						
Russian salad dressing	1 tablespoon							1	
Diet orange soda	1 can								0
Dinner									
Eggplant and tomatoes	1 cup cooked		1						
Olive oil	1 tablespoon							3	
Thin spaghetti	1 cup cooked				2				
Grated parmesan cheese	4 tablespoons						1		
Water	1 cup								
Snacks/desserts									
Hershey Kisses	5								125
Unsalted raw walnut halves	7 (½ ounce)					1		1	
Oreo cookie	1								50
Skim milk	1 cup						1		
Water	2 cups								
Totals for the day	**1**	1.375	1	4	4	2.5	6	225	
Dietary Guidelines goals for the day	**2**	2.5	3	3	5.5	3	6	267	
Total daily physical activity	Circle a 1 for each 10-minute interval completed ① ① ① ① 1 1 1 1 1								

*Discretionary calories should be recorded as calories, not as number of portions.

manner consistent with MyPyramid is to preserve my good health (knock on wood), improve my nutrient intake, and bring more balance to my diet as I maintain my weight. I'm a very active person, although when I'm swamped with work and family commitments, I don't get in as much activity as I'd like. In an ideal week, I do three 30-minute walks on the treadmill (walking about 2 miles per half hour), I take a 1-hour tap dancing class and a 1-hour Pilates class, and I walk a lot outside while running errands, playing with my kids, or simply picking up or dropping off my kids at school (I live and work in New York City, and my kids' schools are within walking distance).

Using the chart from MyPyramid (see page 24), I need about 2,000 calories a day to maintain my weight, based on my gender, age, and activity level. Since my goal is to maintain my weight, I skipped step 4, since 2,000 calories seems to be a good calorie level for me. In step 5, I looked at the meal plan chart (see page 25). A 2,000-calorie meal plan includes:

Fruits: 2 cups

Vegetables: 2½ cups

Grains: six 1-ounce equivalents (at least 3 whole grains)

Meat and beans: 5½ 1-ounce equivalents

Milk: 3 cups

Oils: 27 grams (6 teaspoons)

Discretionary calories: 267 calories

I then recorded these totals for the food groups in the "Dietary Guidelines totals for the day" section of the Daily Food and Fitness Tracker.

If you look at my total intake for one day and compare it with the ideals encouraged by the Dietary Guidelines (step 6), you'll see that I fell short in a few key areas. Of course, this was just one sample day; on other days, I came very close to meeting the goals of the Dietary Guidelines. So I made a list of some ways I could improve my overall nutrient intake, both over the course of one entire day and over the course of a week. Here's what I hoped to achieve during my two-week "trial":

- Increase my fruit intake. How would I do this? I love fruit, especially pink grapefruit sections, bananas, cantaloupe, watermelon, honeydew, and McIntosh apples. But I get lazy, and because I'm not a big snacker, I often turn to nuts or chocolate instead of fruit. So I decided to grab a banana or a cup of fruit salad on my way to work every day and have it between breakfast and lunch. I would try to have banana slices on my cereal at least twice a week. Having 1 cup of fruit or a large banana, which would add to my 1 cup a day of orange juice (I cannot give that up!), would help me meet my 2-cup-a-day quota.

- Increase my vegetable intake. When I have a salad for lunch (about three times a week), it's very easy for me to meet my 2½-cup quota for vegetables. Also, at dinner, I love anything made with tomatoes or eggplant, but I also use red onions when I cook chicken or flank steak fajitas. So I decided that on the days when I didn't have a salad for lunch, I would prepare a baggie with a combination of carrots, cucumbers, and cherry tomatoes to have as a midday snack at my desk. And for dinner, I would be sure to make a vegetable every night that I cooked—potatoes count, too, and I love to make sweet potato French fries and roasted red potatoes (which my kids also love). My goal when eating out was to always order a salad or lightly sautéed vegetables like broccoli or spinach.

- Increase my whole-grain intake. I usually do pretty well with this, especially when I start my day with oatmeal or cereal. My breakfasts vary from day to day, depending on what I'm in the mood for, as well as on what my two small boys want. If they had their way, they'd have pancakes or waffles every day of the week! But I try to mix it up, and we alternate between scrambled eggs with cheese and whole-wheat toast; whole-grain, high-fiber cereal; waffles; and pancakes. I decided that on most days, I would try to knock out two of my three-a-day whole-grain servings by having either whole-wheat toast, oatmeal, or cereal. I would also use whole-wheat breads or flour tortillas for my sandwiches or have brown rice when I order Chinese food for dinner once a week.

- Increase my milk intake. I don't eat yogurt (although I highly recommend it as an excellent vehicle for calcium and protein). So that leaves milk and cheese. As long as I evenly divide my choices between milk and cheese, I can definitely fulfill this quota, though I'll mostly choose full-fat cheeses over lower-fat ones since I prefer the former. I'll also try to consume some other high-calcium foods like broccoli to fill in gaps when I don't have enough cheese or milk. I decided to try to have cereal at least three times a week. I will have some cheese on most days. And on the days when I don't have cereal, I'll make sure to have a glass of milk before bed (this is very easy, especially when I have a cookie). Remember, it's all about balance (and it is only one cookie).

It's been two weeks since I decided to eat more in line with the Dietary Guidelines. While some days have been better than others, I've worked hard toward filling in the nutritional gaps in my diet. Instead of eating pancakes or waffles on most mornings, I now usually alternate oatmeal with cereal, and on the weekend I often have a scrambled egg with cheese and whole-grain bread on one day and pancakes with my kids on the other. My fruit intake has improved, and I'm drinking more milk. I limit my chocolate nibbles to two or three Hershey Kisses a day instead of my usual five or six. I am doing better, and I'm more aware of how to balance out my days in order to take in the most nutrients and still leave some room for higher-fat and/or less nutritious choices that add a little pleasure and enjoyment to life.

With practice and with the help of this book, you'll learn how to follow these basic principles of the Dietary Guidelines:

- Watch your total calorie intake (especially when it comes to "extras" like solid fats, sugary foods, and alcohol).
- Fit more physical activity into your day.
- Fill up on fruits and vegetables.
- Choose whole grains more often than refined ones.
- Opt for leaner cuts of meat.
- Choose low-fat or nonfat milk, cheese, and yogurt more often.

- Steer clear of trans fats.
- Limit sodium intake and reach for high-potassium foods.

If you make all or most of these changes as outlined here, I have no doubt that you'll have a more nutritient-dense, well-balanced diet, yet still be able to choose from a tasty array of foods. You may even find that you're eating more food but, at the same time, taking in fewer total calories. You'll also realize that even some of your favorite treats, like cookies and wine, which contribute calories but few nutrients, can be included in your diet. With just a small commitment of time and a little nutritional know-how, you'll discover that a diet doesn't have to be a temporary form of penance that you go on and off of but instead is part of a healthful lifestyle that you can maintain long term. This new outlook will improve your nutrient intake and overall eating habits and will help you achieve your health-related goals.

3

All Foods Can Fit

There's no need to give up any foods or beverages you enjoy while you incorporate the principles of the Dietary Guidelines into your life. As you'll see in the following pages, no food is off limits. Even your favorites can be included in your custom-fit diet, as long as most of the food choices you make are nutrient-dense. To help you get started, this chapter contains a list of the key food categories encouraged by the new Dietary Guidelines.

The Fruit Bowl

As a general food category, fruit is a major source of vitamins A and C, potassium, fiber, and antioxidants (see "More Than Just Fiber" on page 40), all of which can play a role in preventing or treating type 2 diabetes, heart disease, and cancer. Fruit is high in water content and fills you up with relatively few calories. So not only does fruit add a little sweetness to the diet, but it also packs a nutritional punch.

What Counts as a Fruit?

The fruit category consists of all fresh, frozen, canned, and dried fruits and fruit juices that are in their most basic and nutritious form—they don't contain any added sugars or fats. There are about 60 calories per ½-cup.

More Than Just Fiber

Here are some top fruit bowl picks that pack an antioxidant punch (in order from most to least):

Wild blueberries

Cultivated blueberries

Whole cranberries

Blackberries

Prunes

Raspberries

Strawberries

Red delicious apples

Granny Smith apples

Sweet cherries

Black plums

Plums

Gala apples

Source: Journal of Agricultural and Food Chemistry 52(12), June 9, 2004: 4026–37.

How Much Fruit to Aim for Each Day

In the table below, look for your calorie level and the suggested amount of fruit to aim for each day.

The following count as ½ cup of fruit (see appendix A to find more foods in this category):

- ½ cup of cut-up raw, cooked, or frozen fruit
- 1 medium fruit (for example, an apple, a banana, an orange, a peach, or a pear)
- ½ cup of 100 percent fruit juice (for example, apple juice, cranberry juice, or orange juice)

Suggested Daily Amount (in Cups) for Fruits			
Calorie Level	Amount	Calorie Level	Amount
1,000	1	2,200	2
1,200	1	2,400	2
1,400	1½	2,600	2
1,600	1½	2,800	2½
1,800	1½	3,000	2½
2,000	2	3,200	2½

- ¼ cup of dried fruit (for example, dried apricots, cranberries, currants, dates, figs, peaches, prunes, or raisins)

These fruits are superstars in terms of the following key nutrients:

- Vitamin A: mango, cantaloupe, and apricots (fruits that are bright orange in color)
- Vitamin C: guava, papaya, oranges, and orange juice
- Folate: oranges and orange juice
- Potassium: bananas, plantains, many dried fruits, and oranges

The Vegetable Garden

Vegetables are great sources of vitamins A and C, potassium, fiber, and iron, not to mention antioxidants. They are low in fat and very filling, and many vegetables provide few calories.

What Counts as a Vegetable?

The vegetable group includes all fresh, frozen, and canned vegetables and vegetable juices that are made or prepared without any added sugars or fats.

How Much to Aim For

In the following table, look for your calorie level and the suggested daily amount of vegetables to aim for each day.

Suggested Daily Amount (in Cups) of Vegetables			
Calorie Level	Amount	Calorie Level	Amount
1,000	1	2,200	3
1,200	1½	2,400	3
1,400	1½	2,600	3½
1,600	2	2,800	3½
1,800	2½	3,000	4
2,000	2½	3,200	4

Suggested Weekly Amount (in Cups) for Different Subcategories of Vegetables					
Calorie Level	Dark Green	Orange	Legumes	Starchy	Other
1,000	1	½	½	1½	3½
1,200	1½	1	1	2½	4½
1,400	1½	1	1	2½	4½
1,600	2	1½	2½	2½	5½
1,800	3	2	3	3	6½
2,000	3	2	3	3	6½
2,200	3	2	3	6	7
2,400	3	2	3	6	7
2,600	3	2½	3½	7	8½
2,800	3	2½	3½	7	8½
3,000	3	2½	3½	9	10
3,200	3	2½	3½	9	10

Source: USDA.

In addition to the suggested daily amounts for vegetables, there is a suggested weekly amount for certain subcategories such as dark green vegetables (broccoli, spinach, romaine lettuce, and collard, turnip, and mustard greens) and orange and deep-yellow vegetables (carrots, sweet potatoes, winter squash, and pumpkin). See the table above for the weekly amounts to aim for in each subcategory of vegetables, depending on your calorie level.

How many calories are in ½ cup? The calories within this food group vary, depending on the type of vegetable you select. The following table shows the calories in ½ cup of vegetables.

Approximate Calorie Counts for Vegetables	
Subclass of Vegetables	Calories per ½ Cup
Dark green, deep-yellow, and other vegetables	20 to 30
Starchy vegetables	70
Legumes	115

The following vegetables count as ½ cup (or 1 serving); see appendix A to find more foods in this category:

- ½ cup of cut-up raw or cooked vegetables (including starchy vegetables like potatoes)
- ½ cup of vegetable juice
- 1 cup of leafy salad greens
- ¼ cup of legumes or soybean products (including dried beans and peas, such as pinto beans, kidney beans, lentils, chickpeas, and tofu). Legumes and soybean products may be counted in *either* the meat and beans category or the vegetable category. I recommend that in order to keep within your target calorie level, count legumes often in the meat and beans group if you follow a vegetarian diet or eat a lot of these foods.

The following vegetables are high in the following key nutrients:

- Vitamin A: carrots, sweet potatoes, pumpkin, spinach, collards, and turnip greens
- Vitamin C: broccoli, peppers, tomatoes, cabbage, potatoes, romaine lettuce, turnip greens, and spinach
- Folate: cooked dried beans and peas, spinach, and mustard greens
- Potassium: baked white or sweet potatoes, cooked greens (such as spinach), and winter (orange) squash

Great Grains

The grains group provides complex carbohydrates and key nutrients, including folate, iron, thiamine, niacin, and magnesium. Whole grains are important sources of fiber, as well as of folate, thiamin, iron, and magnesium, while refined grains are lower in fiber but are fortified with folic acid, thiamin, riboflavin, niacin, and iron.

Whole-Grain Options

Amaranth	Triticale
Barley	Wheat berries
Brown rice	Whole-grain barley
Buckwheat	Whole-grain corn
Bulgur (cracked wheat)	Whole Kamut
Graham flour	Whole oats
Millet	Whole rye
Oatmeal	Whole spelt
Popcorn	Whole wheat
Teff	Wild rice

What Counts as a Grain?

Grains include:

- Whole grains: whole-grain products (such as whole-wheat and rye breads, whole-grain cereals and crackers, oatmeal, whole-wheat pasta, and brown rice) and foods made with whole grains.
- Other grains: refined-grain products and foods made with refined grains, such as white breads, enriched-grain cereals and crackers, enriched pasta, and white rice.

How Much to Aim For

In the table on page 45, find your calorie level and the suggested amounts for whole grains and other grains. Try to make whole grains at least half of your grains (the remaining can be other grains).

There are about 80 calories in a 1-ounce equivalent.

The following count as a 1-ounce equivalent (see appendix A to find more foods in this category).

Whole Grains

- 1 cup of ready-to-eat cereal flakes
- ½ cup of cooked oatmeal
- 1 ounce (usually 1 slice) of whole-wheat and rye breads

Suggested Daily Amounts of Grains in 1-Ounce Equivalents		
Calorie Level	Whole Grains	Other Grains
1,000	1½	1½
1,200	2	2
1,400	2½	2½
1,600	3	2
1,800	3	3
2,000	3	3
2,200	3½	3½
2,400	4	4
2,600	4½	4½
2,800	5	5
3,000	5	5
3,200	5	5

- 1 ounce of dry brown rice
- ½ cup of cooked brown rice
- 1 ounce of dry whole-wheat pasta
- ½ cup of cooked whole-wheat pasta
- 1 ounce of whole-wheat crackers (3 to 5 crackers)

Other Grains

- 1 slice of white bread
- 1 cup of cereal flakes made with enriched grains
- 1 ounce of crackers made with enriched grains
- ½ cup of cooked white rice
- 1 ounce of dry pasta
- ½ cup of cooked pasta

Lean on Meats and Beans

Lean meats and beans provide an array of vitamins, including niacin, vitamin B_6, and vitamin E, as well as protein and the mineral zinc. The dried beans and peas (these can also be counted in the vegetable group) provide a lot of fiber.

What Foods Are Included in the Meat and Beans Category?

This category includes meats and poultry in their leanest, most low-fat form (e.g., skinless, white meat chicken), fish, dried beans and peas, eggs, nuts, and seeds.

How Much to Aim for in a Day

Find your calorie level and the suggested daily amount in the table below.

There are about 55 calories per 1-ounce equivalent.

The following count as a 1-ounce equivalent of meat and beans (see appendix A to find more foods in this category):

- 1 ounce of lean meat
- 1 ounce of lean poultry
- 1 ounce of fish, including cod, haddock, and catfish
- 1 egg
- ¼ cup of cooked dried beans
- ¼ cup of tofu

The following count as a 1-ounce equivalent of meat and beans plus 1 teaspoon of oil (see page 50 and appendix A for more about the oil food category):

- 1 tablespoon of peanut butter or almond butter
- ½ ounce of nuts or seeds

Suggested Daily Amounts of Meats and Beans in 1-Ounce Equivalents			
Calorie Level	Amount	Calorie Level	Amount
1,000	2	2,200	6
1,200	3	2,400	6½
1,400	4	2,600	6½
1,600	5	2,800	7
1,800	5	3,000	7
2,000	5½	3,200	7

The following foods are especially high in antioxidants: small red beans, red kidney beans, pinto beans, pecans, and black beans.

Milk, Please

Milk and milk products are important vehicles for key nutrients such as calcium, potassium, vitamin D, and protein. A diet that includes milk and milk products can help lower the risk for low bone mass in people of all ages. Foods in this category include all milks, yogurts, frozen yogurts, dairy desserts, cheeses (except cream cheese), and lactose-free and lactose-reduced products in their lowest-fat forms.

How Much to Aim for in a Day

Find your calorie level and the recommended number of daily milk servings in the table below.

There are about 80 calories in 1 cup of milk, although calories vary. The following count as 1 cup of milk (see appendix A to find more foods in this category):

- 1 cup of skim milk
- 1 cup of nonfat yogurt
- 1½ ounces of natural cheese
- 2 ounces of processed cheese

Suggested Daily Amounts of Milk Products in 1-Ounce Equivalents			
Calorie Level	Amount	Calorie Level	Amount
1,000	2	2,200	3
1,200	2	2,400	3
1,400	2	2,600	3
1,600	3	2,800	3
1,800	3	3,000	3
2,000	3	3,200	3

Approximate Calories for Milk Products		
Milk Product	Approximate Calories	Counts As
1 cup 1% milk	100	1 milk + 20 discretionary calories
1 cup 2% milk	125	1 milk + 40 discretionary calories
1 cup whole milk	145	1 milk + 65 discretionary calories
1 cup low-fat chocolate milk	160	1 milk + 75 discretionary calories
1½ ounces cheddar cheese	170	1 milk + 90 discretionary calories
1½ ounces mozzarella cheese, whole milk	130	1 milk + 45 discretionary calories
1 cup fruit-flavored low-fat yogurt	240–250	1 milk + 100–115 discretionary calories
1 cup frozen yogurt	220	1 milk + 140 discretionary calories
1 cup ice cream, vanilla	290	1 milk + 205 discretionary calories
¼ cup cheese sauce	120	1 milk + 75 discretionary calories

With the exception of fat-free or skim milk, all choices also contribute extra calories, counted as "discretionary calories" (see page 52 for a more complete description of discretionary calories). The table above lists some foods that fall into the milk category but that also contribute discretionary calories.

If you are allergic to milk, don't eat dairy because you don't like the taste, or are lactose intolerant, you can get your calcium from other food sources as shown in the table on page 49.

Oils

Oils are fats that are liquid at room temperature. They come from plant sources and certain fish. Many oils are key sources of vitamin E and monounsaturated and polyunsaturated fatty acids (including the essential fatty acids) in the diet. Oils from plant sources (vegetable and nut oils) contain no cholesterol.

What Foods Are Included in Oils?

This category consists of oils that are added to foods during processing, cooking, and at the table, and the oils found naturally in foods. These include:

Nondairy Food Sources of Calcium*

Food, Standard Amount	Calcium (mg)	Calories
Fortified ready-to-eat cereals (various), 1 ounce	236–1,043	88–106
Soy beverage, calcium-fortified, 1 cup	368	98
Sardines, Atlantic, in oil, drained, 3 ounces	325	177
Tofu, firm, made with calcium, ½ cup	253	88
Pink salmon, canned, with bones, 3 ounces	181	118
Collards, cooked from frozen, ½ cup	178	31
Molasses, blackstrap, 1 tablespoon	172	47
Spinach, cooked from frozen, ½ cup	146	30
Soybeans, green, cooked, ½ cup	130	127
Turnip greens, cooked from frozen, ½ cup	124	24
Ocean perch, Atlantic, cooked, 3 ounces	116	103
Oatmeal, plain and flavored, instant, fortified, 1 packet prepared	99–110	97–157
Cowpeas, cooked, ½ cup	106	80
White beans, canned, ½ cup	96	153
Kale, cooked from frozen, ½ cup	90	20
Okra, cooked from frozen, ½ cup	88	26
Soybeans, mature, cooked, ½ cup	88	149
Blue crab, canned, 3 ounces	86	84
Beet greens, cooked from fresh, ½ cup	82	19
Bok choy, Chinese cabbage, cooked from fresh, ½ cup	79	10
Clams, canned, 3 ounces	78	126
Dandelion greens, cooked from fresh, ½ cup	74	17
Rainbow trout, farmed, cooked, 3 ounces	73	144

Source: Dietary Guidelines for Americans, 2005, 6th Edition, Appendix B-4. Nutrient values from Agricultural Research Service (ARS) Nutrient Database for Standard Reference, Release 17. Foods are from ARS single-nutrient reports, sorted in descending order by nutrient content in terms of common household measures. Food items and weights in the single-nutrient reports are adapted from those in the 2002 revision of USDA Home and Garden Bulletin no. 72, Nutritive Value of Foods.

*Standard amounts listed here are not recommended portions; use your individual meal plan to determine the appropriate portion size of these foods to consume. Mixed dishes and multiple preparations of the same food item have been omitted from this table.

Note: You should consider both calcium content and bioavailability when selecting dietary sources of calcium. Some plant foods have calcium that is well absorbed, but the large quantity of plant foods that would be needed to provide as much calcium as is in a glass of milk may be unachievable for many people. Many other calcium-fortified foods are available, but the percentage of calcium that can be absorbed is unavailable for many of them.

Almond butter

Avocados

Canola oil

Corn oil

Cottonseed oil

Margarine (soft, trans fat–free)

Mayonnaise

Mayonnaise-type salad dressings

Nuts and seeds

Olive oil

Olives

Peanut butter

Peanut oil

Safflower oil

Salad dressings made with vegetable oils

Sesame oil

Soybean oil

Sunflower oil

Walnut oil

How Much to Aim for Each Day

The table below shows the recommended number of grams and teaspoons of oils, based on your calorie level.

There are about 45 calories in one teaspoon.

The following items count as 1 teaspoon of oil (for more foods in this category, see appendix A):

Suggested Daily Amounts (in Grams and Teaspoons) of Oils		
Calorie Level	Grams	Teaspoons*
1,000	15	3
1,200	17	3½
1,400	17	3½
1,600	22	5
1,800	24	5
2,000	27	6
2,200	29	6
2,400	31	7
2,600	34	7
2,800	36	8
3,000	44	9
3,200	51	11

*These are approximate values; each number was rounded down if its value was below ½ and rounded up if its value was above ½. Each teaspoon has approximately 4½ grams.

1 teaspoon of

- Canola oil
- Corn oil
- Cottonseed oil
- Margarine (soft, trans fat–free)
- Mayonnaise (full fat)
- Olive oil
- Peanut oil
- Safflower oil
- Sesame oil
- Soybean oil
- Sunflower oil
- Walnut oil

1 tablespoon of

- Light or low-fat margarine (soft, trans fat–free)
- Light or low-fat mayonnaise
- Most salad dressings
- Peanut butter (also counts as a 1-ounce equivalent of meat and beans)
- Almond butter (also counts as a 1-ounce equivalent of meat and beans)

2 tablespoons of light salad dressing
⅛ small avocado, sliced
15 small black olives, pitted
8 large black olives, pitted
7 green olives (queen size)
12 stuffed green olives
½ ounce (approximately 2 tablespoons) of nuts (also counts as a 1-ounce equivalent of meat and beans)

Salad dressing and olives contain significant amounts of sodium, especially olives (see the sodium content for olives in the following list), so it is recommended that you keep the amounts of these foods small; this is particularly important if you have hypertension or are salt-sensitive. The daily recommended amount of sodium is less than 2,300 mg; for those who have hypertension or are salt-sensitive, the recommendation is less than 1,500 mg.

The following is a list of olives and their approximate sodium content in milligrams:

1 small black olive, pitted	27
1 large black olive, pitted	38
1 stuffed green olive	82
1 green olive (queen size)	110

Peanut butter, almond butter, nuts, and seeds, though counted in the meat and beans group, also contain oil. One tablespoon of peanut butter or almond butter, or ½ ounce of nuts or seeds, should be counted as a 1-ounce equivalent of meat and beans plus one teaspoon of oil.

Use Your Discretion

Discretionary calories reflect the number of calories you have left over after you've selected foods in their most nutrient-dense forms (without added fats or sugars) from all the categories. For example, if you follow a 2,000-calorie food plan, and you consume the allotted daily amounts for all food categories—choose fruits, vegetables, and grains without added sugars and fats, as well as meats and beans in their leanest forms (for example, the leanest meats like skinless chicken, sirloin steak, and fish, and peanut butter without added sugar) and make all of your milk servings (whether from milk, yogurt, or cheese) fat-free—you will have this many discretionary calories each day:

Suggested Daily Amounts of Discretionary Calories			
Calorie Level	Amount	Calorie Level	Amount
1,000	165	2,200	290
1,200	171	2,400	362
1,400	171	2,600	410
1,600	132	2,800	426
1,800	195	3,000	512
2,000	267	3,200	648

If your goal is to lose weight, you may not want to use some or all of your discretionary calories. If your goal is to maintain your weight, you can use these "extra" calories to do the following:

- **Increase the amount of food selected from each food group.** For example, if you follow a 2,000-calorie plan and you are allotted 5½ ounces of meat and beans, you can use some of these "extra" calories to eat more—for example, up to 7 ounces. See the following list to determine how many "extra" calories you can count for each extra portion of food that you consume within each category. The foods listed represent selections from the basic daily meal plan, using the leanest, most nutrient-dense, no sugar–added selections from within each food category. If calorie data is available from the Nutrition Facts panels on particular products, you can use that instead of the approximate amounts in this food group list.

For every ½ cup extra of:	Count as (approximately):
Fruit	60 discretionary calories
Vegetables:	
Dark green, deep-yellow and other vegetables	25 discretionary calories
Starchy vegetables	70 discretionary calories
Legumes	115 discretionary calories

For every 1-ounce equivalent extra of:	Count as (approximately):
Grains (whole grains and other grains)	80 calories
Meat and beans:	55 calories
Nuts, seeds, peanut butter, or other nut butters	100 calories

For every 1-cup equivalent extra of:	Count as (approximately):
Milk (nonfat)	80 calories

For every 1-teaspoon equivalent extra of:	Count as (approximately):
Oils	45 calories

- **Consume foods that are not in the lowest-fat form or that do not contain added sugars.** For example, if you consume low-fat yogurt instead of fat-free yogurt, any additional calories above 80 (the approximate number of calories in 1 cup of skim milk) would count toward your discretionary calorie allotment. Other examples include ground beef that has more than 5 percent fat by weight, poultry with skin, higher-fat luncheon meats, or sausages. Similarly, foods with added sugars (sugars and syrups added to foods and beverages in processing and preparation, *not* the naturally occurring sugars found in fruits or milk) provide discretionary calories.

  For a list of which foods count as "discretionary calories" and how many calories to count them as, see appendix A.

- **Add oil, sugars, or solid fats to foods you're already eating.** For example, each teaspoon of oil or solid fat you consume would count as approximately 45 discretionary calories; similarly each teaspoon of sugar has 16 discretionary calories (or 4 grams of sugar, which has 4 calories per gram). Solid fats include the additional fat in meat and poultry that is eaten either as part of the meat or poultry product or separately (beef fat—tallow or suet, chicken fat, or pork fat [lard]); milk fat (found in whole milk, cheese, and butter); shortenings used in baked products; hard margarines, stick margarine, coconut oil, or palm kernel oil.

- **Consume alcohol.** The table on page 55 shows some basic calorie counts for alcoholic beverages.

To determine how to count some popular mixed meals that contain foods from more than one food category, see appendix A.

Calorie Counts for Alcoholic Beverages			
Beverage	Approximate Calories per 1 Fluid Ounce[a]	Example Serving Volume in Ounces	Approximate Total Calories[b]
Beer (regular)	12	12	144
Beer (light)	9	12	108
White wine	20	5	100
Red wine	21	5	105
Sweet dessert wine	47	3	141
80-proof distilled spirits (gin, rum, vodka, whiskey)	64	1.5	96

[a]Agricultural Research Service (ARS) Nutrient Database for Standard Reference (SR), Release 17 (www.nal.usda.gov/fnic/foodcomp/index.html). Calories are calculated to the nearest whole number per 1 fluid oz.

[b]The total calories and the alcohol content vary depending on the brand. Moreover, adding mixers to an alcoholic beverage can contribute calories in addition to the calories from the alcohol itself.

4

Moving toward a Healthier Weight

The new Dietary Guidelines for Americans, coupled with the MyPyramid Food Guidance System, provide a great starting point if you want to lose weight and keep it off for life. Based on the latest scientific findings about weight management, the guidelines recommend which foods to eat as well as appropriate portion sizes. They also list the amount and the types of physical activity you can engage in each day to achieve and maintain a healthier body weight long term. And while the Dietary Guidelines and the MyPyramid Food Guidance System are not specifically designed to help you lose weight, they *can* help you lose weight and, at the same time, meet your individual nutrient needs to achieve optimal health. Before we begin, here are their key recommendations to guide your weight-management efforts:

- To maintain a healthy body weight: balance the calories you get from foods and beverages with the calories you spend through daily physical activity and exercise.
- To prevent gradual weight gain as you get older: make small cuts in your calorie intake from foods and beverages and increase your physical activity to expend more calories.

For specific populations, the Dietary Guidelines recommend the following:

- For people who need to lose weight: aim for slow, gradual, and steady weight loss by decreasing your calorie intake (while still meeting your nutrient needs) and increasing your physical activity.
- For overweight children: reduce the rate of body weight gain while still allowing for growth and development. Consult a health care provider before placing any child on a weight-reduction diet.
- Pregnant women: ensure the appropriate weight gain as specified by a health care provider.
- Breastfeeding women: losing a moderate amount of weight is safe and does not compromise the weight gain of the nursing infant.

As I pointed out earlier, the great thing about following the new guidelines is that even if you want to lose weight, you won't have to avoid your favorite foods (see "Are These Really No-No Foods?" in chapter 1). You will be able to fill up on lots of healthful foods that are nutrient-dense and relatively low in calories (like fruits and vegetables, whole grains, and low-fat or nonfat dairy products) and still include small portions of more caloric foods (like

Little Losses, Big Gains

Although many people aspire to lose a lot of weight—30, 40, and even 50 or more pounds—studies show that even modest weight losses that are sustained over time can have enormous health benefits. A review of several randomized, controlled clinical trials found that maintaining a modest weight loss (7 to 10 pounds) reduced the incidence of type 2 diabetes in people at high risk for the disease by a whopping 40 to 60 percent over 3 to 4 years (*Annals of Internal Medicine*, 2004;140:951–57). In another study, losing 15 pounds and maintaining that weight loss for 4 years decreased hypertension risk by 21 to 29 percent in overweight middle-aged and older people (*Archives of Internal Medicine*, June 13, 2005; 165(11): 1298–303). The lesson? Losing a little weight and keeping it off can markedly reduce your disease risk and improve your overall health.

nuts and seeds, legumes, and oils), as well as some low-nutrient indulgences (like cake and wine) if you choose to, albeit in smaller portions and perhaps less frequently than you do now. As a result, your new behaviors will be more likely to stick, not just initially but over time. Before you use the Dietary Guidelines to lose weight, however, be sure to consult with a health care provider if you are an overweight adult or child and have a chronic disease and/or are on any medication, to learn how to safely and effectively manage your condition while you lose weight.

Following are some tips to help you succeed at long-term weight loss:

- Set some goals. Having clear and reasonable goals, such as eating a more healthful breakfast or going to the gym more often, is the first step to achieving these goals. Think of your goal as a specific destination; then decide on the best route to get there. That way, you'll easily see when you've taken a wrong turn.

- Make small changes. Instead of attempting a complete diet overhaul, start by making improvements with just one meal. For example, trade in your sugary soda at lunch for a diet soda, use mustard on your sandwich instead of mayo, or have the sandwich your way with all the fixings, but eat just have half of it—and round out the meal with a cup of fruit salad so that you don't leave hungry. When you've mastered one meal, move on to another. Making small, subtle changes in how you eat throughout the day can help you to successfully lose weight.

- Color your world. Loading up on fruits and vegetables can help you lose weight in two key ways. Eating extra servings of fruits and vegetables in place of higher-calorie foods will cut down on your total daily calories (since most fruits and vegetables are low in calories). Fruits and vegetables are also packed with fiber and have a high water content. They can fill you up and leave less room for high-caloric food choices—and that's an added bonus when you're trying to lose weight.

- Measure your success. Whenever you flip on an NBA game, you check who's ahead. Without the score, the game wouldn't be fun. The same is true of goals: you need to know if you're winning, losing, or holding steady. Whether it's with a tape measure, your bathroom scale, the scale at your doctor's or a registered dietitian's office, or a pair of jeans, make it a weekly habit to check in with yourself. I'm not suggesting that you get too attached to the numbers on the scale or the inches on your tape measure, but using these tools can often keep you on track and let you know when you need to steer a different course or switch gears with your diet and exercise plan.

Can a Salad a Day Keep the Pounds at Bay?

It just may, according to a study published in the October 2004 *Journal of the American Dietetic Association*. Subjects who ate a big salad with a little dressing (that contained 100 calories in total) as a first course at lunch consumed fewer total calories over the course of a day compared with people who skipped the salad. The researchers concluded that eating foods that are low in energy density and high in water content as the first course of a meal enhances satiety, or makes you feel more full, which will help you manage your weight.

- Learn from the past. Few people who change their habits succeed on the first, the second, or even the third try. In fact, behavioral research suggests that it takes at least half a dozen attempts—and often far more—to instill a new habit. If you have a strong sense of self, you will view unsuccessful attempts not as failures but as teachable moments that will help you learn what didn't work, set more reasonable goals, and find new ways to achieve them.

- Get support. Surround yourself with people who support your weight-loss efforts, such as a spouse, a friend, a colleague, a relative, or just someone who shares your goals for healthful eating and increased physical activity. Having support from others and limiting your contact with people who try to sabotage you in any way can help you stay motivated.

- Think ahead. When you change your diet and your activity level, try to make changes that you can maintain not only for a few weeks or months but for the rest of your life. Chances are, if the new habits you practice while you lose weight are similar to those you will incorporate into your lifestyle after you've achieved your goal, you'll be more successful at maintaining your weight loss.

- Fuel your body frequently. There is no magic number for how many times you should eat over the course of the day to lose weight and keep it off long term. Perhaps you don't like to or are unwilling to eat first thing in the morning, or your schedule requires that you eat dinner at midnight. Whatever your situation, a good rule of thumb is to try to eat when you're hungry and don't to go too long in between meals and snacks. This will ward off feelings of starvation that might tempt you to overeat. Keep a variety of healthful snacks like fresh fruit and unsalted nuts or seeds in your bag or briefcase for times when it's tough or impossible for you to eat a balanced meal. These strategies can help you consistently fuel your body (and keep your metabolism revved up so that you're an efficient fat-burning machine), and they'll ward off hunger and supply much-needed nutrients.

- Plan for plateaus. Everyone has them. You lose weight, you feel really great about your appearance and your accomplishment, and then it stops. You're still eating less and moving more, you're doing everything right, but the scale won't budge. Or, you see the pounds creeping up. A plateau is perfectly normal and often occurs after six months of steady weight loss (if not sooner). But a plateau doesn't mean you should stop doing what you're doing. This is the time for you to either eat more frequently (perhaps you're going too long without food between meals) or add a few extra calories (which will inspire your body to burn more calories and may just be what you need to boost your metabolism). Or maybe you're eating more and need to keep a record for a few days or a week or two to get back on track. On the exercise front, you can step up your physical activity—use a different machine at

Can Artificial Sweeteners Make Me Gain Weight?

People often use artificially sweetened foods in an attempt to save calories, but, according to some recent research, that can potentially backfire. A study published in the July 2004 *International Journal of Obesity* found that eating artificially sweetened foods may disrupt the body's natural ability to use taste to judge how many calories a food or a beverage contains. In this study, one group of rats was fed a sugar-sweetened solution, while another group received an inconsistent diet—sometimes the sugar-sweetened solution and sometimes a solution that contained saccharine, an artificial sweetener. After ten days, the rats were able to eat what they wanted, and the rats that were fed both the sugary and the artificially sweetened solutions consumed three times as many calories as did the rats fed the sugar-sweetened solution. The researchers concluded that while artificial sweeteners may promote weight loss if they help you consume fewer calories, they may also confuse your body. Thus, you'll still need to watch your total calorie intake when you consume artificially sweetened foods.

the gym, try a new class, or walk a little faster on the treadmill. If all else fails, it may mean that your body has reached a comfortable weight. Even though it may not be your dream weight, if you can't lose anymore weight despite your best efforts (and there's no medical reason for this such as a thyroid problem that's just kicked in), perhaps you should pat yourself on the back for losing weight in the first place and instead shift your focus toward maintaining the weight loss. You can always revisit the idea of losing weight after a few weeks or months or consult a registered dietitian to discuss other ways to break your plateau.

- Give yourself some wiggle room. After you've lost weight and are at or near your desired goal, give yourself a weight range to stay within. I personally have found this to be an effective strategy for keeping weight off long term. I play around with 2 pounds, and when I'm at my high weight, I step up the physical activity and make some calorie cuts. When I'm down, I admit that I may have that extra Oreo cookie. As long as I give myself that little bit of wiggle room, it helps me enjoy what I'm eating and how I'm moving my body and also provides me with a tangible way to measure how I'm doing.

Here are some painless food substitutions you can make to cut calories (and still preserve taste!).

Tips on Cutting Calories When You Buy or Cook Foods

Instead Of	Choose
The milk group:	
Evaporated whole milk	Evaporated fat-free (skim) or reduced-fat (2%) milk
Whole milk	Reduced-fat (2%), low-fat (1%), or fat-free (skim) milk
Ice cream	Sorbet, sherbet, low-fat, or fat-free frozen yogurt
Whipped cream	Whipped cream made with skim milk or low-fat vanilla yogurt
Sour cream	Plain low-fat yogurt
Cream cheese	Neufchatel or "light" cream cheese or fat-free cream cheese
Cheese	Reduced-calorie or low-calorie cheese
Regular (4%) cottage cheese	Low-fat (1%) or reduced-fat (2%) cottage cheese
Whole milk mozzarella cheese	Part–skim milk, low-moisture mozzarella cheese
Whole milk ricotta cheese	Part–skim milk ricotta cheese
Coffee cream (half and half)	Low-fat or reduced-fat milk or nonfat dry milk powder
Nondairy creamer	Low-fat or reduced-fat milk or non-fat dry milk powder

The grain group:

Bagel	English muffin
Granola	Low-fat granola, bran flakes, cooked grits, or oatmeal

The meat and beans group:

Cold cuts or lunch meats	Low-fat cold cuts (95 to 97 percent fat-free lunch meats, low-fat processed meats)
Hot dogs	Low-fat hot dogs
Bacon or sausage	Canadian bacon or lean ham
Regular ground beef	Extra-lean ground beef, such as ground round (the label should say at least "90% lean"), ground turkey, or ground chicken
Chicken or turkey with skin	White meat chicken or turkey without skin
Duck or goose	White meat chicken or turkey without skin
Oil-packed canned tuna	Water-packed canned tuna (rinse it to reduce the sodium)
Beef (chuck, rib, brisket)	Beef (round eye, top round, bottom round, round tip, top loin, top sirloin, chuck shoulder, and arm roasts), trimmed, and choose select grades
Pork (spareribs, untrimmed loin)	Pork loin, tenderloin, center loin, lean ham
Frozen breaded fish or fried fish	Fish or shellfish, unbreaded (fresh, frozen, canned in water)
Whole eggs	Egg whites or egg substitutes
Frozen dinners (with more than 13 g fat per serving)	Frozen dinners with less than 13 grams of fat per serving

Other tips for meat and beans:

• Trim visible fat from meats and poultry before cooking.

• Broil, grill, roast, poach, or boil meat, poultry, or fish instead of frying.

• Drain off fat that appears during cooking.

• Skip or limit the breading on meat, poultry, or fish, as it adds fat and calories.

• If you choose to bread meat, poultry, or fish, bake it instead of frying it, since the food will soak up more fat when it's fried.

• Prepare dried beans and peas without added fats.

• Limit high-fat sauces or gravies, and instead use spices and low-sodium seasonings to enhance flavor (see "Fill-Ins for Flavor" on page 65).

The oils group:

Regular trans fat–free margarine	Light spread margarines or diet margarines, in a tub, squeeze bottle, or spray bottle
Regular mayonnaise	Light or diet mayonnaise or mustard
Regular salad dressings	Reduced-calorie or fat-free salad dressings, lemon juice, or plain, herb-flavored, or wine vinegar
Vegetable oils	Nonstick cooking spray

Source: Adapted from Clinical Guidelines on the Identification, Evaluation, and Treatment of Overweight and Obesity in Adults: The Evidence Report, *NIH Publication No. 98-4083, September 1998, National Institutes of Health.*

Do you know that old saying "You can lose weight if you eat less and exercise more"? There's certainly a grain of truth in that idea, but making it a reality is hard. It's easy to lose weight on most weight-loss diets, but it's difficult to maintain a healthy weight, especially without regular exercise. This fact may be why the Dietary Guidelines place such an emphasis on physical activity. They encourage more physical activity than ever before—up to 90 minutes a day—because they recognize the key role that physical

Fill-Ins for Flavor

Use these flavorings to replace salt in recipes for meat dishes.

Lean meats: bay leaves, caraway seeds, chives, mustard, lemon juice, garlic, curry powder, onion, paprika, parsley, sage, thyme, allspice, turmeric

Veal: thyme, mace, curry powder, nutmeg

Lamb: basil, curry powder, dill, mace

Lean pork: thyme, savory, rosemary, sage

Poultry: rosemary, nutmeg, mustard, lemon juice, ginger, dill, curry powder, bay leaves

Lean ground meats: allspice, basil, mustard, savory

Lean meat loaf: rosemary, nutmeg

activity plays (of course, in conjunction with improved food choices) in maximizing health. Here's what they recommend:

If your goal is to:	Then do this on most or all days:
Reduce your risk of chronic diseases and improve your quality of life	At least 30 minutes of moderate physical activity
Maintain a healthy body weight and/or prevent unhealthful weight gain	60 minutes of moderate to vigorous physical activity
Maintain your weight after weight loss	At least 60 to 90 minutes of moderate physical activity

Note: Moderate activity is defined as the equivalent of walking about 3.5 miles per hour. Vigorous activity is defined as the equivalent of walking about 4.5 miles per hour. It's important not to exceed calorie intake requirements as well.

The guidelines also recommend the following for special populations:

- *Children and adolescents.* Engage in at least 60 minutes of physical activity on most, and preferably all, days of the week.
- *Pregnant women.* If there are no medical or obstetric complications, do 30 minutes or more of moderate-intensity physical

activity on most, if not all, days of the week. Avoid activities that carry a high risk of falling or abdominal trauma, such as skiing.

- *Breastfeeding women.* Be aware that neither acute nor regular exercise adversely affects the mother's ability to breastfeed.
- *Older adults.* Participate in regular physical activity to reduce functional declines associated with aging and to achieve other benefits of physical activity identified for all adults.

I'm the first to admit that these are lofty goals for physical activity. I hope you don't let these big numbers—30 to 90 minutes a day—scare you off and send you straight to the sofa. While I fully support these science-based physical activity recommendations, I encourage you to think of them as ideals to aspire to, not as something that you absolutely have to achieve.

If you're already exercising and meeting the new guidelines, kudos to you. But if you're doing less than what's recommended, as many of us are, and you want to burn more calories, improve your appearance, build muscle, or achieve any of the health benefits that physical activity and exercise confer, I will now help you overcome your excuses, better manage your schedule, and turn these recommendations into achievable habits.

You can take the following steps to get started. Read through all the steps thoroughly before beginning any exercise program, especially if you are older and/or have any chronic health conditions.

1. **Keep tabs.** On a weekend, write down your upcoming weekly schedule, including all work, family, and other commitments. This is a great way to see where you are in terms of physical activity. Maybe you already go to the gym once or twice a week. Putting pen to paper and seeing your schedule in front of you is a great way to plan how, when, and where you will fit in any additional exercise or activities. Pencil in some time— even 20 minutes, on two separate days—that you will do something, anything, to meet your daily exercise quota.

2. **Create an action plan.** Once you've zeroed in on when you will fit in some physical activity and on what days, think about what kind of activity you would like to do or would

realistically be able to do. If you're at work, can you go to the company gym? Can you take a short walk during your lunch hour? Will you get out of the elevator before your floor and walk up several flights to your office? Will you go to the gym before work for a real wake-up call? Or maybe there's a great class you've been dying to take. For me, it was tap dancing, and over a year ago I found an adult class in my neighborhood. It's the most fun I've ever had exercising. If you can, exercise at the time of day when you feel most energetic. If you're a morning person, exercise when you wake up. If you follow a consistent workout schedule, your body's hormones adjust so that you train most efficiently and with the least fatigue at that particular time of day. Having a plan of action—knowing what you'll do and when you'll do it—can definitely help you incorporate more activity into your day. After all, if you know where you're going, you'll know when you've arrived!

3. Make a list. Write down any and all physical activities you do each day. When I first moved to New York City almost fifteen years ago, I didn't do much formal exercise. So I began to jot down what I did each day, whether I walked outside or on a treadmill, lifted light weights, or went ice skating. For years I've kept a record of my physical activity, and this has motivated me (especially since I can see the progress I've made). You, too, can keep track of your fitness activities—10 minutes at a time. At first, use your Daily Food and Fitness Tracker (see page 22) to add up how many 10-minute bouts of activity you accumulate over the day. In addition to this, you can use the "Fitting in Fitness Worksheet" on page 68 to chart your progress. I suggest that you fill this in before you get started on any exercise program, using your own ideas as well as some of the tips provided in this chapter.

4. Get a buddy. Studies have shown that people who have support from others are more likely to keep exercising. If you'd rather exercise with someone to socialize (and to reduce boredom), ask a coworker, a colleague, a friend, your spouse, a significant other, or even one of your kids to join you. If no one is interested, join a walking club, a bowling league, a running

Fitting in Fitness Worksheet

Fill this in every two weeks or as often as needed to motivate and inspire yourself to stay on track with your physical activity.

Activities I enjoy	Where I call/go for information about this activity	When I plan to engage in this activity	How long I will participate in this activity each day (minutes)	How long I will participate in this activity each week (minutes)
1.				
2.				
3.				
4.				
5.				

Weekly goals:

Did I achieve my weekly goals?

Goals for next week:

club, or some other group that engages in regular enjoyable physical activity. Having support from others can motivate and inspire you to be physically active (not to mention that it will help you make a new friend or two).

5. Set a goal. I was never a runner but started running—albeit very slowly—when I was newly married and first moved to New York City in the early 1990s. To keep myself motivated, I signed up for a 5-kilometer women-only race (about 3.1 miles) on Long Island. Before race day, I had run a few times a week but only 2 miles at a time. On race day (a Sunday morning), my husband and I got up early and headed for Long Island. Needless to say, I had knots in my stomach. When I crossed the finish line, I felt great—and so accomplished. After that, my husband and I joined the New York City Road Runners Club, and my claim to fame, to this day, is that I completed a 10-mile race (though it did take me almost two hours to finish). I don't run now, but I am so proud of my accomplishment. I know that setting goals like completing that race was a great motivator for me. And while you don't have to run in a race, just think about other ways to fit more physical activity into your life—for example, by taking part in five charity walks a year, running 2 miles at a stretch, or walking faster. These are small goals, and if you set your mind to it, you can achieve them. Setting small, attainable goals can be a great motivator—plus, you can always change your fitness goals to accommodate new interests and pursuits.

6. Play it safe. If you plan to exercise on a bicycle, make sure to wear a helmet, reflectors, and other appropriate gear. If you walk or run where there are cars, you might want to leave your music player at home and listen for traffic (here's where having a friend join you comes in handy—you can walk and talk). Be sure to speak with a health care provider to help you design a safe and individualized physical activity program if any of the following special circumstances apply to you: if you have a chronic health problem such as heart disease, hypertension, diabetes, osteoporosis, asthma, or obesity or are at high risk for heart disease—for example, you have a family history of

heart disease or stroke, eat a diet high in saturated fat, trans fats, and cholesterol; or if you're a man over the age of 40 or a woman over the age of 50 and plan to start vigorous physical activity.

7. Think progress, not perfection. This may be the most important step. Many people think that if they can't spend a lot of time doing physical activity (like 60 minutes) or can't work out at least five days a week, that doing less would be a waste of time. Not true. Studies show that even several small bursts of physical activity—just 10 minutes at a time—can add up in terms of health benefits. And, in my opinion, going to the gym twice a week, consistently, is better than going often for a month or two and then stopping cold. Of course, if you make more opportunities to be physically active on a regular basis, you'll enjoy more health and other benefits. But less is certainly better than none when it comes to exercise.

Following are some tips to help keep you safe and motivated:

- Check with your doctor. Your bones may ache, your heart may beat too fast, or you might have some other excuse not to exercise. Discuss exercise with your health care provider before you start—perhaps he or she will give you an individualized exercise prescription. Keep in mind that many physical ailments can improve with activity.

- Don't use age as an excuse. There are people from 90 to 100 years old who compete in the Masters Games, and if you go to a health club, you'll see a lot of gray heads among the treadmill users. Even if it's only a walk, you're not too old to exercise. Regular physical activity is a great way to keep your muscles and body working well and to minimize the decline in function that inevitably occurs as we age.

- Beat your fatigue. One of the best ways to prevent fatigue is by engaging in activities that get your blood and heart going, feed your brain oxygen, and strengthen your muscles. Early or midday exercise can help boost your energy level and can help you fall asleep faster and sleep more soundly at night.

- Do what you love. If you can afford to join a gym and you enjoy going, that's great. But if your idea of exercise isn't walking on a treadmill, find a sport you enjoy, such as tennis or swimming, or take a dance or fitness class, either private or group. It's crucial to make exercise something you like doing; otherwise, you'll dread making it a part of your life. If you enjoy solo activities such as skiing, biking, or running, choose those activities over class-based workouts. Every few weeks or months, vary your activity. This will work different muscle groups and will also keep your activity fresh (and prevent boredom) so that you'll stay motivated and inspired to continue your efforts. Be sure to include some cardiovascular or aerobic exercise (such as walking, running, or swimming), weight training (with light weights, fitness machines, or fitness bands), and stretching to keep yourself limber.

How to Move More at Work (without Losing Your Job!)

- Walk to work, or get off the bus or subway a few stops early and walk the rest of the way.
- Skip the elevator and take the stairs up to your office. If you work on a high floor, get off five floors early and take the stairs.
- Instead of sending an e-mail, get up from your desk and go see your colleague.
- Walk to get your lunch instead of having it delivered.
- Drink a lot of water (then you'll have to get up a lot to go to the bathroom).
- During your lunch break, take a short walk or go to the gym by yourself or with a friend.
- Try some deskercise! You can stretch, do neck rolls or abdominal crunches, and even lift light weights (like the stapler) while sitting at your desk.
- Ask your boss about a worksite wellness program, or start your own fitness group.
- Participate with coworkers as a team in fitness walks for charitable organizations.

- Reward yourself. Is there something you wish to buy or a place you want to visit? Every month (or as often as you need to and as your budget will allow), be sure to reward yourself for accomplishing your fitness goals.
- Distract yourself. Whether it's music, television, or books on tape, having a distraction can really help you get through your workout and can make time pass more quickly. Just be sure to be safe, especially if you plan to walk on the streets or in a park where there is traffic.
- Take a look at yourself. Take your picture once a month and put it on the refrigerator. Keep your targets at the top of your mind by putting sticky notes of your biggest goals on your computer or bathroom mirror.

The bottom line is that balancing calorie intake through better food choices with energy expenditure through regular, consistent, and enjoyable daily physical activity is the best recipe you can use to improve your overall health, maintain feelings of well-being, and manage your weight. If you take small steps and make realistic changes in your diet and fitness habits that will fit into your life, you'll reap many rewards.

5

Picks and Pitfalls
of the Market

If you want to follow the U.S. Dietary Guidelines and select healthful foods at your supermarket, you have to be prepared not only to read labels and check your shopping list but to resist the temptations laid before you by master marketers.

Are you aware that every day you are influenced to make food or beverage choices by their placement in television shows or films you watch? Perhaps one of your favorite desperate housewives was enjoying a certain brand of soda, or a bag of name-brand potato chips sat on her kitchen counter. While you may not realize why you selected these items at the supermarket, food and beverage manufacturers believe that you were influenced by what you saw on television the day or the night before. They're willing to pay product-placement specialists more than $60,000 each time a food or a beverage appears in a scene. Manufacturers would never spend that kind of money if product placement didn't influence shoppers.

Advertising doesn't affect only grown-ups who have money to spend; it has an even greater effect on children. Does your child beg you to buy a certain breakfast cereal after seeing it in a commercial or being eaten by a favorite TV character or movie star? According to Democratic senator Tom Harkin, who recently spoke before a conference of the American Advertising Association, corporate America spends $12 billion a year on advertising to children "because that advertising works brilliantly." He added, "It persuades children to demand—to the point of throwing a tantrum, if necessary—a regular diet of candy, cookies, sugary cereals, and sodas."

Supermarket Strategy

Consider what you see as you push your cart around the supermarket aisles. The items that the store wants to sell you are placed at eye level. The staples you may really need are placed on the bottom or the top shelves.

There is also a phenomenon known as "slotting." Paying for shelf space has become part of the everyday cost of doing business for thousands of grocery stores and their suppliers. With fees ranging as high as $25,000 per item, an estimated $9 billion in slotting fees is paid annually. The average supermarket carries 30,000 different products, out of 100,000 different products to choose from. Because 4 of every 5 of the estimated 15,000 products introduced each year fail, there is a strong desire on the part of manufacturers and retailers to reduce risks. Added to this picture is the low profit margin of the supermarkets.

When you go to the supermarket, therefore, you encounter another form of subliminal mind manipulation—the words that are used to promote certain products. Signs proclaiming "New" or "4 for $4," for example, are commonly used to encourage you to purchase particular items.

It's an undeniable fact that supermarkets are designed to make us buy things. The science of supermarket design is widely practiced with the intent of guiding you to purchase not only as much as possible, but the specific products the supermarket wants you to buy. From the product positioning on shelves to the layout of the store, every effort is made to control your behavior as a shopper.

So if you really want to buy more of the most nutrient-packed foods that are encouraged by the Dietary Guidelines—fruits and vegetables, whole grains, low-fat dairy foods, and lean meats and beans—and less of the fatty, salty, and sugary foods that contain few nutrients and a lot of calories, you must not only be knowledgeable about nutrition, but also be mindful of (and somewhat resistant to) the many subtle influences around you that affect your shopping habits. One great way to do this is to stick to your list. At the end of this chapter, you'll find the Ultimate Grocery Store Shopping List, a complete list you can take along whenever you go food shopping. It's broken down by food group (for example, fruits, vegetables) and includes all the foods, beverages, and other ingredients you'll find in the two-week meal plans in chapter 7, as well as for the recipes in this book. You can photocopy this list and highlight the items you plan to buy, or else add your own items, depending on your weekly menu and to accommodate your own particular choices. But before you run to the grocery store with list in hand, it's important that you learn how to read a food label. This will arm you with great information and the know-how to make more healthful food selections.

The Food Label

Today's food labels provide you with

- Nutrition information about almost every packaged or processed food you'll find in a grocery store.
- A distinctive, easy-to-read Nutrition Facts panel that enables you to quickly find the information you need to make healthful food choices.
- Information on the amount per serving of saturated fat, trans fat, cholesterol, sodium, and other nutrients of major health concern.
- Nutrient reference values, expressed as % Daily Values, that help you see how a specific food fits into your overall daily diet.
- Uniform definitions for terms that describe a food's nutrient

Nutrition Facts

Serving Size 1 cup (236ml)
Servings Per Container 1

Amount Per Serving	
Calories 120	Calories from Fat 45
	% Daily Value*
Total Fat 5g	8%
Saturated Fat 3g	15%
Trans Fat 0g	
Cholesterol 20mg	7%
Sodium 120mg	5%
Total Carbohydrate 11g	4%
Dietary Fiber 0g	0%
Sugars 11g	
Protein 9g	17%

Vitamin A 10%	Vitamin C 4%
Calcium 30% • Iron 0% • Vitamin D 25%	

*Percent Daily Values are based on a 2,000 calorie diet. Your daily values may be higher or lower depending on your calorie needs.

content—such as "light," "low-fat," and "high-fiber"—to ensure that such terms mean the same for any product on which they appear.

- Standardized serving sizes that make nutritional comparisons of similar products easier.

The food label is a key tool for locating and evaluating the nutritional content of the foods and beverages you purchase. The nutrition information has been required on almost every foodstuff since the middle of the 1990s. It provides very valuable information but can be somewhat confusing. Following are explanations that will make the labels clearer and more useful for you.

Daily Values (DV)

The Daily Values consist of two sets of references for nutrients:

- Daily reference values (DRVs)
- Reference daily intakes (RDIs)

Daily Reference Values (DRVs)

These designations are for nutrients for which no set of standards previously existed, such as fat, cholesterol, carbohydrates, proteins, and fibers. DRVs for these energy-producing nutrients are based on the number of calories consumed per day. For labeling purposes, 2,000 calories has been established for calculations. This level was chosen, in part, because many health experts say it approximates the maintenance calorie requirements of the group most often targeted for weight reduction: postmenopausal women.

DRVs for the energy-producing nutrients are calculated as follows:

- Fat is based on 30 percent of calories.
- Saturated fat is based on 10 percent of calories.
- Carbohydrates are based on 60 percent of calories.
- Protein is based on 10 percent of calories.
- Fiber is based on 11.5 grams of fiber per 1,000 calories.

The DRVs for cholesterol, sodium, and potassium, which do not contribute calories, remain the same no matter what the calorie level.

Because of the links between certain nutrients and specific diseases, DRVs for some nutrients represent the uppermost limit considered desirable. Eating too much fat or cholesterol, for example, has been linked to heart disease, and eating too much sodium, to the risk of high blood pressure. Therefore, the label shows you that a product has less than the uppermost limits of DRVs for fats, cholesterol, and sodium, which are

- Total fat: less than 65 g
- Saturated fat: less than 20 g
- Trans fat: counted as part of saturated fat (so aim for less than 20 grams of saturated fat and trans fat combined)
- Cholesterol: less than 300 mg
- Sodium: less than 2,400 mg

Reference Daily Intakes (RDIs)

This is a set of dietary references based on and replacing the recommended dietary allowances (RDAs) for essential vitamins and minerals and, in select groups, protein. You will continue to see vitamins and minerals expressed as percentages on the label, but these figures now refer to the daily values.

The following table shows the RDIs—once familiar to us as RDAs, based on the National Academy of Sciences 1968 recommended dietary allowances:

Nutrient	Amount
Vitamin A	5,000 International Units (IU)
Vitamin C	60 milligrams (mg)
Thiamin	1.5 mg
Riboflavin	1.7 mg
Niacin	20 mg
Calcium	1.0 gram (g)
Iron	18 mg
Vitamin D	400 IU
Vitamin E	30 IU
Vitamin B_6	2.0 mg

Nutrient	Amount
Folic acid	0.4 mg
Vitamin B_{12}	6 micrograms (mcg)
Phosphorus	1.0 g
Iodine	150 mcg
Magnesium	5 mg
Copper	2 mg
Biotin	0.3 mg
Pantothenic acid	10 mg

The mandatory and voluntary dietary components on the label and the order in which they must appear are

- Total calories
- Calories from fat
- Calories from saturated fat (including trans fats)
- Stearic acid (on meat and poultry products only)
- Polyunsaturated fat
- Monounsaturated fat
- Trans fat
- Cholesterol
- Sodium
- Potassium
- Dietary fiber
- Soluble fiber
- Insoluble fiber
- Sugars
- Sugar alcohol (for example, the sugar substitutes xylitol, mannitol, and sorbitol)
- Other carbohydrates (the difference between total carbohydrates and the sum of dietary fiber, sugars, and sugar alcohol, if declared)
- Protein
- Vitamin A

- Percentage of vitamin A present as beta-carotene
- Vitamin C
- Calcium
- Iron
- Other essential vitamins and minerals.

If a food is fortified or enriched with any of the optional components, or a claim is made about any of them, pertinent additional nutrition information becomes mandatory. These mandatory and voluntary components are the only ones allowed on the nutrition panel.

When a caloric value for a serving of food is less than 5 calories, the FDA allows the label to read "zero" calories. If the fat calories are less than 0.5 grams, it can read "zero calories from fat."

Label Lingo

The following is a list of some common terms on food labels and what they mean.

Term	Definition
Low calorie	Fewer than 40 calories per serving.
Low sodium	140 mg or less per serving.
Very low sodium	Less than 35 mg per serving.
Sodium free	Less than 5 mg per serving.
Low fat	3 g or less per serving.
Low saturated fat	1 g or less per serving.
Low cholesterol	20 mg or less per serving.
High or source of	Denotes the beneficial presence of a nutrient such as fiber or vitamins.
High or excellent source of	Contains 20 percent or more of the daily value (see page 76) for a particular nutrient in a serving.
Good source of	Supplies 10 to 19 percent of the daily value (see page 76) for a particular nutrient.

Term	Definition
Reduced	Means that a product has been nutritionally altered and contains at least 25 percent less of a nutrient (such as fat) or 25 percent fewer calories than the regular product.
Less	Means that a product contains 25 percent less of a nutrient or 25 percent fewer calories than the reference food. For example, pretzels that have 25 percent less fat than potato chips could carry a "less" claim.
Light or lite	Signifies that a product contains ⅓ fewer calories or ½ the fat of the comparison food. "Light in sodium" may be used on food in which the sodium content has been reduced by at least 50 percent.
More	Means that a product contains at least 10 percent more of the daily value (see page 76) for a desirable nutrient, such as fiber, than the regular food.
Fresh	Signifies a food that has not been heat processed or frozen and supposedly contains no preservatives.
Lean and extra lean	Describes the fat content of meats, poultry, seafood, and game meats. Lean = less than 10 g fat per serving. Extra lean = less than 5 g fat per serving.
Percent fat free	Used only to describe foods that qualify as low fat.
High potency	Describes a nutrient in a food that is 100 percent or more of the RDI (see page 77) established for that product; the term may also be used with multi-ingredient products if two-thirds of the nutrients are present at 100 percent of the RDI.

| Antioxidant | May be used in conjunction with currently defined claims for "good source" and "high" to describe a nutrient scientifically shown to be absorbed in a sufficient quantity, such as vitamin E, to inactivate free radicals or prevent free radical-initiated chemical reactions in the food. |
| Low carb | Officials at the U.S. Food and Drug Administration haven't yet set a definition of low carb, reduced carb, or carb light. |

Here's a primer to use when you're navigating through your local supermarket aisles to help you find products made with whole grains and those that provide less sodium, added sugar, fat, and cholesterol.

Going for the Grain

If you're trying to bump up your whole-grain intake, learning to translate the lingo on food labels and ingredients lists when you compare products will make it that much easier. Following are some tips:

- Read the ingredient list on the food label. For many whole-grain products, the words *whole* or *whole grain* will appear before the grain ingredient's name. The whole grain should be the first ingredient listed. The following are whole grains:

    Brown rice

    Bulgur

    Graham flour

    Oatmeal

    Whole-grain corn

    Whole oats

    Whole rye

    Whole wheat

    Wild rice

- Wheat flour, enriched flour, and degerminated cornmeal are *not* whole grains. And foods labeled with the words *multigrain*, *stone-ground*, *100% wheat*, *cracked wheat*, *seven-grain*, or *bran* are usually *not* whole-grain products (bran, though only part of the whole grain, does provide health benefits).

- Look for the whole-grain health claim—*"Diets rich in whole-grain foods and other plant foods and low in total fat, saturated fat, and cholesterol may help reduce the risk of heart disease and certain cancers"*—on food product labels. Foods that bear the whole-grain health claim must contain 51 percent or more whole grains by weight and be low in fat.

- Color is not an indication that a product is a whole grain or is made with whole grains. Bread can be brown because of molasses or other added ingredients. Read the ingredient list to see whether it is a whole grain.

- Use the Nutrition Facts panel to compare products. Choose those that have a higher percent daily value (%DV) for fiber—the %DV of fiber is a good indication of the amount of whole grain the product contains.

The following table shows what to look for on bread, cereal, or cracker labels:

When You Buy:	Look For:
Bread (1 ounce/1 slice)	• A whole grain listed as the first ingredient • Less than 3 grams of fat • At least 3 grams of fiber • Zero trans fats (less than 0.5 gram per serving)
Ready-to-eat cereal (1 ounce)	• A whole grain listed as the first ingredient • Less than 3 grams of fat • Less than 10 grams of sugar • Zero trans fats (less than 0.5 gram per serving)

Crackers (1 ounce)
- A whole grain listed as the first ingredient
- Less than 3 grams of fat
- At least 3 grams of fiber
- Zero trans fats (less than 0.5 gram per serving)

Finding the Sodium

Sometimes, you have to read between the lines to understand food labels. Certain terms on packages may be misleading. *Unsalted, processed without salt,* or *no salt added* may signify that the producer didn't put in any additional salt during processing, but the food may still be naturally high in sodium. For example, a low-sodium soy sauce has 390 milligrams of sodium per teaspoon (and who can use only one teaspoon of soy sauce on a dish?) and a popular tomato-vegetable drink with "no salt added" has 90 milligrams of sodium per 4.5 fluid ounces. Salt can also be listed under dozens of "sodium" designations, such as monosodium glutamate and sodium caseinate, adding even more salt to your diet.

The following tips will help you identify lower-sodium food choices and reduce your daily intake of sodium to less than 2,300 milligrams per day (less than 1,500 milligrams a day if you have been diagnosed with hypertension or are salt-sensitive):

- Look for labels that say *low sodium, very low sodium,* or *sodium free.*
- Most of the sodium in the food supply comes from packaged foods. Processed meats such as hams, sausages, frankfurters, and luncheon or deli meats are particularly high in sodium. Make these "once-in-a-while" foods to keep your sodium intake (not to mention your intake of saturated fat and cholesterol) in check.
- Fresh chicken, turkey, and pork that have been enhanced with a salt-containing solution also have added sodium. Check the product label for statements such as "self-basting" or "contains up to ___% of ___."
- Frozen dinners, packaged mixes, cereals, cheese, breads,

soups, salad dressings, and sauces also tend to be high in sodium. The amounts in different types and brands often vary widely, so be sure to read labels and compare.

• Choose fresh, plain frozen, or canned vegetables without added salt most of the time.

• Choose fresh or frozen fish, shellfish, poultry, and meat most often. They are lower in salt than most canned and processed forms.

• Ask your grocer or supermarket to offer more low-sodium foods.

When you cook or prepare food at home, you can make these flavorful substitutions for salt:

Salt Substitutions

Food	Alternative Flavoring
Lean meats	Bay leaves, caraway seeds, chives, mustard, lemon juice, garlic, curry powder, onion, paprika, parsley, sage, thyme, allspice, turmeric
Veal	Thyme, mace, curry powder, nutmeg
Lamb	Basil, curry powder, dill, mace
Lean pork	Thyme, savory, rosemary, sage
Poultry	Rosemary, nutmeg, mustard, lemon juice, ginger, dill, curry powder, bay leaves
Lean ground meats	Allspice, basil, mustard, savory
Lean meat loaf	Rosemary, nutmeg
Stews	Allspice, bay leaves, onion, sage, caraway seeds, basil
Soups	Thyme, savory, parsley, paprika, onion, basil, chives, curry powder, dill, garlic, bay leaves
Breads	Caraway seeds, nutmeg (toast), sage (biscuits), rosemary (stuffing), cinnamon, mace

Salads	Basil, dry mustard, savory, caraway seeds, chives, cider vinegar, garlic, lemon juice, dill, paprika, parsley, pimiento, onion, thyme
Fruit	Almond extract, ginger, cinnamon (especially apples), nutmeg, peppermint extract, mace, allspice (especially in peaches, applesauce, and cranberry sauce)
Vegetables	Lemon juice, chives, dill, cider vinegar, pimiento, parsley, dry mustard, garlic, mace, onion, paprika
Tomatoes	Allspice, bay leaves, curry powder, garlic, dill, thyme, savory, sage
Potatoes	Nutmeg, mace, garlic, dill, rosemary
Onions	Thyme, sage
Green beans, lima beans, or peas	Savory, sage, rosemary, thyme
Pie crust	Nutmeg, cinnamon
Puddings	Peppermint extract, almond extract, nutmeg
Mayonnaise	Curry powder, dry mustard

Finding the Hidden Sugar

Labels can be confusing when it comes to sugar as well. A food can be labeled "sugar free" or "sugarless" and still contain calories from sugar alcohols such as xylitol, sorbitol, and mannitol. To limit added sugars, as called for in the Dietary Guidelines, read the food label's ingredient list. Look for the following terms on ingredient lists. They add up to one thing—sugar:

Brown sugar	Fruit juice concentrate
Corn sweetener	Glucose
Corn syrup	High-fructose corn syrup
Dextrose	Honey
Fructose	Invert sugar

Lactose	Raw sugar
Maltose	Sucrose
Malt syrup	Syrup
Molasses	Table sugar

Let's take good old apple pie, as an example of how you can read a food label to find hidden sugar. The ingredient list is usually located under the Nutrition Facts panel or on the side of a food label. Ingredients are listed in order by weight. The ingredient in the greatest amount by weight is listed first and the one in the least amount is listed last. For example, in the following ingredient list, corn syrup is the second ingredient listed and sugar is the third, which means that, combined, these two sugars are the main ingredients in the apple pie.

Baked Apple Pie

Ingredients: Apples, corn syrup, sugar, water, modified corn starch, dextrose, brown sugar, sodium alginate, spices, citric acid, salt, dicalcium phosphate. In a pastry consisting of enriched bleached wheat flour (niacin, reduced iron, thiamine mononitrate, riboflavin, folic acid), vegetable shortening (partially hydrogenated soybean and/or cottonseed oil), water, sugar, less than 2 percent of salt, yeast, l-cysteine (dough conditioner), lecithin.

Steering Clear of Fat, Saturated Fat, Trans Fats, and Cholesterol in Food

The new Dietary Guidelines call for 20 to 35 percent of your total calories from fat, with less than 10 percent of your total calories from saturated fat, to keep dietary cholesterol to less than 300 mg a day, and to have as little trans fat as possible. The following tips will help you buy foods to lower your intake of saturated fat, trans fats, and dietary cholesterol.

- Choose vegetable oils or trans fat–free soft margarine, rather than solid fats (such as shortening, butter, and hard margarine). Read labels and compare.

- Buy the leanest cuts of meat (see chapter 4), including lean ground beef.
- Buy skinless chicken breasts.
- Limit your intake of high-fat processed meats, such as bacon, sausages, salami, bologna, and cold cuts, and look for lower-fat versions as alternatives.
- Buy egg substitutes as an alternative to eggs.
- Choose fat-free or low-fat milk, yogurt, and cheese.
- Consume most of your fats from sources of polyunsaturated and monounsaturated fatty acids, such as fish, nuts, and vegetable oils.
- Choose fewer foods made with saturated fats and trans fats.

The Top Sources of Saturated Fat, from Most to Least

- Cheese
- Beef
- Milk
- Oils
- Ice cream/sherbet/frozen yogurt
- Cakes/cookies/quick breads/doughnuts
- Butter
- Other fats (such as shortening and other animal fats)
- Salad dressings/mayonnaise
- Poultry
- Margarine
- Sausage
- Potato chips, corn chips, popcorn
- Yeast bread
- Eggs

**The Top Sources of Trans Fats
from Most to Least**

- Cakes, cookies, crackers, pies, bread, etc.
- Animal products
- Margarine
- Fried potatoes
- Potato chips, corn chips, popcorn
- Household shortening
- Breakfast cereals, candy, and other sources

What about Those Health Claims?

Health claims characterize a relationship between a substance (a specific food or a food component) and a disease or a health-related condition. An example of an authorized health claim, which by definition must contain the elements of a substance and a disease, is *"Calcium may reduce the risk of osteoporosis"* (or also *"Yogurt, a calcium-containing food, may reduce the risk of osteoporosis"*). While the FDA has not issued a regulation for a health claim for a specific food (for example, a banana, which is a "substance" that can be consistently characterized), with adequate evidence such a health claim could be authorized.

The established health claims for foods for a number of years have been

- Calcium and osteoporosis
- Fat and cancer
- Saturated fat and cholesterol and coronary heart disease
- Fiber-containing grain products, fruits, and vegetables and cancer
- Fruits, vegetables, and grain products that contain fiber, particularly soluble fiber, and coronary heart disease
- Sodium and hypertension
- Oats and oat flour and cholesterol

The FDA is reviewing all qualified health claims before they are used on food labels. This process involves a full review of the available scientific evidence and may include a detailed assessment by experts on scientific evidence affiliated with the Agency for Healthcare Quality Research or by other independent experts, in addition to FDA staff, as appropriate. The FDA also announced it will work closely with the Federal Trade Commission (FTC), the agency that helps to regulate advertising.

One of the first health claims made under the new rules is that walnuts can help ward off heart disease. Similar claims for other nuts are cracking the health-labeling barrier.

The new Dietary Guidelines will go far toward making you an informed consumer and will recommend healthful foods to help you create a dietary plan that's right for you. Whether your goal is to eat more nutritiously, manage your weight, or manage or prevent diet-related diseases, you need to understand what you're up against in the supermarket. If you know how to read a food label and have a shopping list in hand, you can personalize the Dietary Guidelines to fit your life.

The Ultimate Grocery Store Shopping List for the New Dietary Guidelines

On the following pages I have provided a comprehensive shopping list that includes spaces in each category for you to write in additional food items you enjoy. Before you fill in the blanks, think about what you'll need to feed yourself and your family during the upcoming week. You can copy this list and place it on your refrigerator or kitchen bulletin board as a reminder of what to buy.

The Ultimate Grocery Store Shopping List

Fruit
Fresh Fruit

- ❏ Apples, green
- ❏ Apricots
- ❏ Avocados*
- ❏ Bananas
- ❏ Blackberries
- ❏ Blueberries
- ❏ Cantaloupe
- ❏ Cherries, sweet
- ❏ Currants
- ❏ Grapefruit, pink
- ❏ Grapes—red, green
- ❏ Honeydew
- ❏ Kiwifruit

- ❏ Mandarin oranges
- ❏ Mangoes
- ❏ Oranges
- ❏ Peaches
- ❏ Pears
- ❏ Plums
- ❏ Raspberries
- ❏ Star fruit
- ❏ Strawberries
- ❏ Watermelon
- ❏ _____
- ❏ _____
- ❏ _____

*Avocados are technically fruits, but because of their high monounsaturated fat content, they count toward your oil intake.

Canned Fruit (in juice or water)

- ❏ Natural applesauce
- ❏ Olives—black, pitted, canned*
- ❏ _____

- ❏ _____
- ❏ _____
- ❏ _____
- ❏ _____

*Olives are technically fruits, but because of their high monounsaturated fat content, they count toward your oil intake.

Frozen Fruits (without added sugar)

- ❏ _____
- ❏ _____

- ❏ _____
- ❏ _____

Dried Fruit (without added sugar)

- ❏ Dried apricots
- ❏ Dried cranberries
- ❏ Raisins
- ❏ _____

- ❏ _____
- ❏ _____
- ❏ _____
- ❏ _____

100% Fruit Juices
- ❏ Orange juice
- ❏ _____
- ❏ _____
- ❏ _____

Other
- ❏ Apple butter
- ❏ _____
- ❏ _____
- ❏ _____

Vegetables
Fresh Vegetables (or packaged fresh)

- ❏ Arugula
- ❏ Asparagus
- ❏ Bamboo shoots
- ❏ Basil
- ❏ Bay leaves
- ❏ Bibb lettuce
- ❏ Broccoli
- ❏ Brussels sprouts
- ❏ Cabbage
- ❏ Cauliflower
- ❏ Carrots, whole, baby, shredded
- ❏ Celery
- ❏ Cucumbers
- ❏ Dill
- ❏ Eggplant—Italian, Japanese
- ❏ Garlic, cloves
- ❏ Green beans
- ❏ Mushrooms—shitake, portobello
- ❏ Onions—red and white
- ❏ Parsnips
- ❏ Parsley
- ❏ Peppers—red and green
- ❏ Potatoes—red, baby creamer, russet
- ❏ Pumpkin
- ❏ Red leaf lettuce
- ❏ Romaine lettuce
- ❏ Scallions
- ❏ Shallots
- ❏ Squash, spaghetti, butternut
- ❏ Spinach salad
- ❏ Swiss chard
- ❏ Tomatoes—yellow, red, and cherry
- ❏ Turnips
- ❏ Zucchini
- ❏ _____
- ❏ _____

Canned Vegetables *(make most of your choices low-sodium or no salt added and no sugar added)*

- ❑ Corn
- ❑ Pumpkin
- ❑ Sun-dried tomatoes, packed in oil (count as oil because of high oil content)
- ❑ Tomatoes

- ❑ Tomato puree
- ❑ Tomato sauce
- ❑ _____
- ❑ _____
- ❑ _____
- ❑ _____

Frozen Vegetables *(without added fats)*

- ❑ _____
- ❑ _____

- ❑ _____
- ❑ _____

Beans and Legumes

- ❑ Black beans, canned (low-sodium or no salt added)
- ❑ Kidney beans, canned (low-sodium or no salt added)
- ❑ Lentils—French green, red
- ❑ Soy crumbles
- ❑ Soy milk, vanilla

- ❑ Tofu, made with calcium
- ❑ Vegetable burgers (from Boca Burger or Morning Star Farms)
- ❑ Vegetarian refried beans
- ❑ _____
- ❑ _____
- ❑ _____
- ❑ _____

Grains

Breads, Rolls, Mixes

- ❑ Flour tortillas—whole wheat, white
- ❑ Kaiser rolls
- ❑ Pancake and waffle mixes
- ❑ Whole-wheat bread
- ❑ Whole-wheat English muffins
- ❑ Whole-wheat hamburger buns

- ❑ Whole-wheat pitas
- ❑ Whole-wheat rolls
- ❑ Whole-wheat waffles
- ❑ _____
- ❑ _____
- ❑ _____
- ❑ _____

Cereals

- ❏ Corn flakes
- ❏ Granola cereal, low-fat (no added raisins)
- ❏ Grape Nuts cereal
- ❏ Kellogg's Special K cereal
- ❏ MultiGrain Cheerios
- ❏ Oat bran flakes

- ❏ Oatmeal
- ❏ Oats, rolled
- ❏ _____
- ❏ _____
- ❏ _____
- ❏ _____

Crackers

- ❏ Graham crackers
- ❏ Whole-grain crackers
- ❏ Whole-wheat crackers
- ❏ _____

- ❏ _____
- ❏ _____
- ❏ _____

Rice

- ❏ Brown rice
- ❏ Wild rice
- ❏ Spanish rice
- ❏ _____

- ❏ _____
- ❏ _____
- ❏ _____
- ❏ _____

Pasta

- ❏ Bow tie
- ❏ Gemelli
- ❏ Penne, whole wheat
- ❏ Spaghetti

- ❏ _____
- ❏ _____
- ❏ _____
- ❏ _____

Other Grains, Snacks

- ❏ Bread crumbs
- ❏ Cornmeal, yellow degerminated
- ❏ Couscous
- ❏ Croutons
- ❏ Flour—white, whole wheat
- ❏ Matzo meal
- ❏ Matzo ball soup mix, Manischewitz

- ❏ Popcorn—unsalted, bagged, kernels
- ❏ Pretzel rods
- ❏ Tortilla chips, blue corn
- ❏ Wheat germ
- ❏ Whole-wheat pretzels
- ❏ _____
- ❏ _____
- ❏ _____
- ❏ _____

Milk

Milk
- ❏ Fat-free (skim) milk
- ❏ Low-fat (1%) buttermilk
- ❏ Low-fat (1%) milk
- ❏ _____

- ❏ _____
- ❏ _____
- ❏ _____

Yogurt
- ❏ Low-fat yogurt—plain, vanilla, lemon, blueberry
- ❏ Nonfat yogurt, vanilla
- ❏ _____

- ❏ _____
- ❏ _____
- ❏ _____

Cheese (natural, fresh, processed)
- ❏ American cheese—full-fat, reduced-fat, low-fat
- ❏ Cheddar cheese—shredded or solid, low-fat
- ❏ Mozzarella cheese, fresh
- ❏ Parmesan cheese, grated
- ❏ Swiss cheese—reduced-fat, reduced-sodium

- ❏ Cottage cheese—low-fat, reduced-fat, fat-free
- ❏ Feta cheese
- ❏ Gouda, smoked
- ❏ _____
- ❏ _____
- ❏ _____
- ❏ _____

Other
- ❏ Frozen yogurt, any flavor
- ❏ Ice cream, any flavor
- ❏ Pudding cups or mix, any flavor

- ❏ _____
- ❏ _____
- ❏ _____
- ❏ _____

Meats and Beans

Meats
- ❏ Beef—lean, ground
- ❏ Flank steak
- ❏ Chicken breast—boneless, skinless
- ❏ Chicken—lean, ground
- ❏ Chicken—whole

- ❏ Chicken sausage, Italian
- ❏ Pork chops
- ❏ Turkey—fresh roasted, deli (lower-fat, lower-sodium), ground

- ❑ _____
- ❑ _____

- ❑ _____
- ❑ _____

Fish

- ❑ Cod fish
- ❑ Crab
- ❑ Salmon
- ❑ Tuna—chunk white light, canned, packed in water

- ❑ _____
- ❑ _____
- ❑ _____
- ❑ _____

Beans (see "Vegetables")

Nuts, Nut Butters, and Seeds (Raw, Dry Roasted, Unsalted)

- ❑ Almond butter
- ❑ Almonds—shaved, whole
- ❑ Cashews
- ❑ Peanuts
- ❑ Peanut butter, natural (no added sugar)
- ❑ Pine nuts

- ❑ Sesame seeds
- ❑ Walnuts—chopped, whole
- ❑ _____
- ❑ _____
- ❑ _____
- ❑ _____

Eggs

- ❑ Large eggs
- ❑ Egg substitute

- ❑ _____
- ❑ _____

Oils

- ❑ Margarine, soft tub with no trans fats
- ❑ Mayonnaise, light
- ❑ Oil—canola, olive, peanut, safflower, sesame (roasted)
- ❑ Olive oil spray
- ❑ Salad dressing—Caesar, Italian, Ranch (reduced-fat, low-fat, creamy)

- ❑ _____
- ❑ _____
- ❑ _____
- ❑ _____
- ❑ _____

Condiments, Spices, and Seasonings

- ❑ Bacon bits
- ❑ Bouillon, chicken
- ❑ Cayenne pepper
- ❑ Chili powder
- ❑ Cilantro
- ❑ Coriander
- ❑ Cumin
- ❑ Cinnamon
- ❑ Ginger root
- ❑ Honey mustard
- ❑ Ketchup
- ❑ Lemon juice
- ❑ Mustard, yellow
- ❑ Nutmeg
- ❑ Oregano
- ❑ Parsley
- ❑ Red pepper flakes
- ❑ Rosemary
- ❑ Soy sauce, low-sodium
- ❑ Tarragon leaves, dried
- ❑ Teriyaki sauce, light
- ❑ Vietnamese chili garlic sauce
- ❑ Vinegar—apple cider, balsamic
- ❑ _____
- ❑ _____
- ❑ _____
- ❑ _____

Other Foods (solid fats, sugary foods or foods with added sugars, alcoholic beverages, baking items, miscellaneous)

- ❑ Almond biscotti
- ❑ Baking powder (aluminum-free, if possible)
- ❑ Brown sugar
- ❑ Cocoa powder
- ❑ Coconut, shredded
- ❑ Chocolate syrup
- ❑ Chocolate chip cookies
- ❑ Cream cheese—light, whipped
- ❑ Dessert pops, frozen
- ❑ Jelly beans
- ❑ Maple syrup, light
- ❑ Nonstick cooking spray
- ❑ Spanish sherry
- ❑ Sugar—cane, powdered
- ❑ Vanilla extract
- ❑ Wine—red, white
- ❑ _____
- ❑ _____
- ❑ _____
- ❑ _____

Beverages

- ❑ Coffee
- ❑ Iced tea, unsweetened
- ❑ Water, carbonated, bottled
- ❑ _____
- ❑ _____
- ❑ _____
- ❑ _____

Miscellaneous

❑ _____   ❑ _____

❑ _____   ❑ _____

❑ _____   ❑ _____

❑ _____

6

Dining Out without Giving In

It's one thing to eat a balanced and nutritious diet in our own homes. Yet it's much more difficult to make healthful food and beverage choices when we are out in the real world. When we step beyond our front doors, the proliferation of fast foods, convenience meals, and out-of-control portions makes it hard to resist temptation.

But don't despair. You don't have to stay home to make smart, sensible food choices. Using the new guidelines and the tips in this book, you'll learn how to navigate unscathed through fast-food places, food courts, delis, airport snack bars, and your local takeout restaurant. You'll even be able to enjoy gourmet upscale restaurants without regret. Your new dietary plan will stay intact because, after you read this chapter, you'll know how to make more healthful choices whenever and wherever you eat.

Fast Food

While many fast-food restaurants continue to expand their portion sizes and increase their high-calorie, high-fat offerings (think of Hardee's Monsterburger and Burger King's Enormous Omelet Sandwich), some fast-food giants have stepped up to the plate to offer low-fat milk (McDonald's), as well as fresh fruit cups and low-fat yogurt (Wendy's). Even though the nutritional pickings are

Can Fast Food Make You Fat?

We all know that fast food provides fast calories, mainly from fat. But did you know that even a few weekly visits to the drive-thru can, over time, catch up with you and contribute to the development of obesity and type 2 diabetes? A study published in the January 1, 2005, *Lancet* found a strong link between fast-food consumption and weight gain and insulin resistance in both black and white adults ages 18 to 30. People who ate fast food more than twice a week gained 10 pounds more and had twice the rate of insulin resistance, compared with those who had fast food less than once a week. The bottom line? Think of fast food as a once-in-a while treat, not a daily or a weekly habit.

slim, fast food doesn't have to mean fast calories if you eat small portions and try to make more healthful selections.

Following are some tips for eating fast food:

- Choose white meat chicken breast over fried, breaded white, or dark meat chicken.
- Look for restaurants that make hamburgers out of lean 100 percent ground beef.
- Choose grilled meats over breaded and fried ones.
- Have it your way: ask for your burger or grilled chicken sandwich without mayonnaise or without cheese (or with only one slice); add your own light mayonnaise or mustard.
- Ask for nutritional information so that you know what you're eating.
- Order child-sized portions of hamburgers, side dishes, and beverages.
- Eat only in clean-looking restaurants. If a restaurant or its employees do not appear clean, chances are the food isn't clean either.

Better fast-food bites include:

- A plain hamburger with lettuce, tomato, mustard, or ketchup
- A grilled chicken breast sandwich without mayonnaise

- A garden salad with reduced-fat dressing
- Low-fat or nonfat yogurt or frozen yogurt
- Whole-grain cereal with low-fat milk
- A fresh fruit cup

A Healthful Head Start: Best Bets for Breakfast

Breakfast is one of the best times to eat whole grains, fruits, and milk, three of the food groups encouraged in the new Dietary Guidelines. Having a nutrient-packed start to your day can give you energy to perform better, both mentally and physically. Following are some sample combinations that you will likely find at most eating venues. They are packed with fiber, calcium, and other vital nutrients that your body and brain need to thrive. These combinations work great in the morning but can be eaten at lunch or dinner, too.

- Fresh pineapple chunks mixed with low-fat cottage cheese and a slice of whole-wheat toast with apple butter
- A whole-wheat English muffin topped with soft margarine and a hard-boiled egg
- Whole-grain or bran cereal with low-fat or skim milk and shaved almonds, served with a piece of fresh fruit
- Oatmeal topped with a sprinkle of brown sugar and walnut halves
- An egg-white omelet loaded with peppers and low-fat cheddar cheese in a toasted whole-wheat pita pocket and served with low-fat milk
- Multigrain pancakes or waffles topped with banana slices
- Nonfat yogurt topped with low-fat granola and dried apricots

At a Deli or Sandwich Bar

If you find yourself opting often for a traditional sandwich for lunch, the following tips will help you build a better sandwich:

- Order sandwiches made on whole-wheat bread.
- Ask for less meat (2 to 4 ounces should be plenty, depending on your individual calorie needs).
- Ask for vegetable toppings like lettuce, tomato, peppers, grilled vegetables, or a small amount (⅛) of a small avocado.
- Ask for sides of condiments like mayonnaise (light or regular) or salad dressing and apply them yourself.
- Order a half sandwich and a small cup of vegetable-based soup, such as minestrone.
- Order a bean-based soup as a main course.
- Round out your meal with a banana, an apple, or any fresh fruit, or opt instead for a fresh mixed-fruit cup

The Perfect Snack

Whether you're traveling, running errands, or sitting at a desk all day, knowing what to grab when the midafternoon munchies strike cannot only help you meet your nutrient needs, but also give you energy and prevent you from raiding your friend's candy dish or grabbing a sugary drink from a vending machine or a gas station. Following are some key foods that you can mix and match, depending on your personal preferences. They will provide calories to give you energy, protein and fiber to sustain you, and a healthful dose of unsaturated fats to add taste and flavor. To save time, fill a few small bags so that you'll have something easy to stash in your purse or briefcase or grab when you're on the go. Pick one food from each category, and keep the calories between 200 and 300 per bag.

1. Meat and beans: unsalted, dry roasted, or raw nuts—cashews, peanuts, almonds, walnuts, sunflower seeds

2. Grains: low-fat granola cereal (without raisins) or any whole-grain crunchy cereal

3. Fruits: dried fruit such as raisins, apricots, cherries, cranberries, bananas, pineapple, and dates (choose those without added sugar)

Raising the Bar with Your Salad

Whether it's a help-yourself salad bar or one where someone makes a salad with ingredients you choose, here are some tips to pack the most taste and punch into your salad. With everything that's in it, a salad truly eats like a meal!

- Choose one of the following lettuces: spinach, romaine, or mixed field greens (about 2 cups total).
- Choose two or more of the following colorful vegetables: tomatoes, carrots, green beans, peppers, onions, or cucumbers (about 1 cup total).
- Choose two of the following lean meats and/or beans: tuna, roasted turkey, grilled chicken, chickpeas, tofu, kidney beans, or other beans (about three 1-ounce equivalents in total).
- Choose one of the following cheeses: shredded cheddar, crumbled feta cheese, or fresh mozzarella (about 1 ounce total).
- Choose one or more of the following to top your salad: vinaigrette or any low-fat salad dressing (about 2 tablespoons); mustard, lemon juice, and light mayonnaise may also be used or combined to make a salad dressing.
- Choose one of the following to accompany your salad: green or red grapes, green apple slices, dried apricots or raisins, or another dried fruit (about 2 tablespoons).

The amounts of each item will vary, depending on your individual calorie needs and food preferences (see chapter 2).

Top Tips to Play It Safe When You Eat Out

Following are some general tips to help you make better food choices and create more well-rounded meals when you eat out:

- Make the vegetables fill about half of your plate. Think of them as the stars of the meal, and use equal portions of meat or beans and starch or grains as the supporting players.

- Round out your meal with a beverage. Some more healthful alternatives to sugary soda and fruit drinks include plain water, seltzer with or without a slice of lemon or lime, a spritzer (made with half fruit juice and half sparkling water), unsweetened iced tea, low-sodium tomato or vegetable juice, unsweetened tea, 1% or skim milk, or any other beverage with no added sugar.

- For a two-course meal, start with a vegetable soup or a garden salad with a side of oil and vinegar; ask for the dressing on the side and use your fork to dip into it.

- When you order beef, poultry, fish, or other meats, ask for them broiled, steamed, or grilled; limit dishes in which the meats are fried or heavily sautéed.

Reading between the Lines

To save calories and fat when you place your order, look for terms on the menu such as:

steamed	poached
in its own juice (au jus)	tomato juice
garden fresh	dry broiled (in wine or lemon
broiled	juice)
baked	lightly sautéed
roasted	stir-fried

instead of terms like:

butter sauce	marinated (in oil)
fried	stewed
crispy	basted
creamed	sautéed
in cream or cheese sauce	stir-fried
au gratin	casserole
au fromage	hash
escalloped	prime
parmesan	pot pie
hollandaise	pastry crust
béarnaise	

- Keep your eye on portion size. Ask for smaller portions when you choose main dishes, side dishes, and beverages; for example, see if the restaurant can serve you a half order of pasta.
- When you can, skip the buffet and order directly from the menu. If you don't have a choice, take one lap around the buffet to see what's available; then fill up one plate and one plate only.
- Ask your waiter to remove the bread or chip basket from the table once you (and others at your table) have had enough.
- If the main course you receive is much larger than you anticipated, eat half and ask the waiter to wrap up the other half for you to take home.
- Taste each bite of food, and stop when you're full (even if your plate's not empty).
- If dessert is a must, choose fruit or sorbet or have just a bite or two of cake (save more than this for a special occasion).

Finally, when you're at a restaurant, ask a lot of questions and ask for what you want. Your waiter will probably want to help you order what you like so that you enjoy your dining experience, so ask and you may very well receive!

Following are some of the better choices among a variety of ethnic cuisines, whether you're eating at a restaurant or ordering takeout.

Chinese

Even though many of the offerings at Chinese restaurants are fried, greasy, or loaded with fat (think egg rolls, shrimp rolls, and spareribs), there are many healthful selections to choose from. While it's prudent to avoid or limit salty sauces (especially if you have high blood pressure or are salt-sensitive) or to ask for less sauce or sauce on the side from which you can dip, eating Chinese food is a great opportunity to get an array of vegetables and whole grains into your diet.

At a Chinese restaurant (or when you order takeout), look for foods that are:

- Steamed
- Jum (poached)
- Chu (boiled)
- Kow (roasted)
- Shu (barbecued)

Choose foods made with or cooked in:

- Hoisin sauce (used to flavor assorted Chinese vegetables, including broccoli, mushrooms, onions, cabbage, snow peas, scallions, bamboo shoots, water chestnuts, and asparagus)
- Oyster sauce (made from seafood)
- Mild sauce (foods that are lightly stir-fried)
- Light wine sauce
- Hot and spicy tomato sauce
- Sweet and sour sauce
- Hot mustard sauce
- Reduced-sodium soy sauce

Choose dishes that are:

- Made without monosodium glutamate (MSG)
- Garnished with spinach or broccoli

Choose more of these items:

- Fresh fish filets, shrimps, scallops
- Chicken, without skin
- Lean beef
- Bean curd (tofu)
- Moo shu vegetables, chicken, or shrimp
- Steamed brown rice
- Lychee fruit

French

Butter? Steak? Egg dishes? Fatty sauce? What's not to like? Although many dishes at French restaurants are loaded with fat and cholesterol, there are also wonderful salads, grilled lean meats, and seafood dishes from which to choose. Usually, portions are small, so that can be helpful if you're watching your waistline.

At a French restaurant, try to choose these foods more often:

- Dinner salad with vinegar or lemon juice dressing (or another reduced-fat dressing)
- Vegetable soup
- Top loin (strip) or tenderloin (with sauce on the side, if desired)
- Fresh grilled fish, shrimps, scallops, or steamed mussels (without creamy sauces)
- Grilled chicken breast (skinless)
- Fresh fruit for dessert

Italian

Who doesn't love the cheesy, oily, meaty comfort food provided by an Italian restaurant? If you overdo the cheesy or creamy sauces, you're bound to consume too many calories and too much total fat and saturated fat. But if you make more healthful selections and keep your portions small, eating Italian food can help you meet your daily and weekly quotas for vegetables and beans.

Choose dishes that are grilled, lightly sautéed, or made with:

- Onions
- Shallots
- Peppers and mushrooms
- Artichoke hearts
- Red sauces such as a spicy marinara sauce (*arrabiata*) or cacciatore
- Light red or white wine sauce
- Light mushroom sauce
- Red clam sauce
- Lemon sauce
- Capers
- Herbs and spices such as garlic and oregano

- Crushed tomatoes and spices
- Spinach (*Florentine*)
- Lemon (*piccata*)

Some healthful Italian fare includes:

- Mozzarella, tomato, and basil salad
- Garden salad with Italian dressing
- Minestrone
- Pasta e fagioli (pasta, beans, and tomatoes in broth)
- Fish with fresh vegetables

Middle Eastern

Eating Middle Eastern food is a great way to incorporate a variety of seasonings, spices, and unique flavors into your diet. Many of the dishes contain beans and vegetables, which will help you get your quota of these high-nutrient foods.

Choose dishes made with:

- Lemon dressing or lemon juice
- Middle Eastern spices
- Other herbs and spices
- Mashed chickpeas
- Fava beans
- Smoked eggplant
- Tomatoes, onions, green peppers, and cucumbers
- Spiced garlic sauce
- Spiced ground meat
- Chopped parsley and onions
- Couscous, rice, or bulgur (cracked wheat)

Choose dishes that are:

- Basted with tomato sauce
- Stuffed with rice and imported spices
- Grilled on a skewer
- Marinated and barbecued

- Baked
- Charbroiled or charcoal broiled

Japanese

Although some dishes are fried or prepared with a lot of fat, Japanese food offers many soups, vegetables, and dishes made with seafood, tofu, and other soybean products. If you're watching your sodium intake, remember to steer clear of sauces (or ask for lower-sodium options).

Choose these more often:

- House salad with fresh ginger and cellophane (clear rice) noodles
- Rice
- *Nabemono*, a quick-cooked stew
- Chicken, fish, or shrimp teriyaki
- *Menrui*, or soba noodles, often used in soups
- Broiled foods (*yakimono*)
- Tofu, or bean curd
- Grilled vegetables

Indian

Eating Indian food is a tasty way to incorporate some unique flavors (not to mention yogurt and beans) into your diet.

Choose these more often:

- Baked unleavened bread
- Masala
- Tandoori
- Paneer (a delicate cottage-type cheese)
- Lentils, chickpeas (garbanzo beans), beans
- Potatoes
- Basmati rice (*pullao*)
- *Matta* (peas)
- Chicken or shrimp kebabs

Choose foods that are cooked with

- Yogurt
- Green vegetables, onions, tomatoes, peppers, and mushrooms
- Spinach (*saag*)
- Curry
- Dried fruits (often used as a garnish)

Mexican

As long as you don't go overboard on chips and salsa early on, eating Mexican food can please your palate with a variety of spices and unique flavors. Although some of the dishes are fried and way too cheesy, Mexican fare can include loads of fresh or lightly sautéed vegetables, beans, lean meat, and fish, as well as a variety of grains.

Choose these more often:

- Grilled meat or fish
- Shredded spicy chicken
- Rice and black beans
- Shrimp or chicken fajitas
- Fish marinated in lime juice and mixed with spices (*ceviche*)

Choose foods that are made or served with:

- Salsa (hot red tomato sauce)
- Salsa verde (green chili sauce)
- Enchilada sauce
- Shredded lettuce, diced tomatoes, and onions
- Corn or soft wheat tortilla
- Chili vegetarian tomato sauce
- Picante sauce

Thai

Feeling hot hot hot? Thai foods offer a variety of unusual fruits, vegetables, and rice seasoned with herbs and spices to fire you up. If you're watching your cholesterol, make sure not to order too many dishes made with coconut (it's high in saturated fat). Otherwise, eat up!

Choose foods that are:

- Barbecued
- Lightly sautéed
- Broiled
- Boiled
- Steamed
- Braised
- Marinated
- Charbroiled

Choose foods made or served with:

- Basil sauce, basil, or sweet basil leaves
- Lime sauce or lime juice
- Chili sauce or crushed dried chili flakes
- Thai spices
- Pineapple (hollowed-out)
- Fish sauce
- Hot sauce
- Napa, bamboo shoots, black mushrooms, ginger, or garlic
- A bed of mixed vegetables
- Scallions, onions

Steakhouses

Usually, you can get a variety of salads and steamed or lightly sautéed vegetables, baked potatoes, and grilled seafood dishes, in addition to lean meats like sirloin, at most steak restaurants. Beware, however, of the fried and greasy accompaniments and the delectable desserts; if you choose to have these, make the portions small.

Choose these more often:

- Lean broiled beef (3 to 6 ounces), such as London broil, filet mignon, sirloin, and round and flank steak
- Tomato and onion salad, chopped salad, or garden salad with balsamic vinaigrette

- Green beans, spinach, or broccoli, steamed or lightly sautéed in olive oil and garlic (and/or lemon juice and herbs)
- Grilled or baked fish or other seafood dishes

Portion Sizes

How often do you eat out or order in? If you are like most Americans, you average 4.2 such meals per week, according to a recent National Restaurant Association report. You may eat more or fewer meals that are made outside your home, but the reality is that, according to the USDA, foods cooked in a commercial kitchen tend to contain more fat and saturated fat, as well as less calcium, fiber, and iron, compared with foods you prepare at home. The portions also tend to be bigger when you eat out. The table below shows just a few examples of how portion sizes have changed over the last two decades.

Clearly, you face many obstacles to eating well when you eat out. Yet, the information in this book and in the new Dietary Guidelines and the MyPyramid Food Guidance System will help you make more healthful menu choices whenever you dine in restaurants, eat on the run, grab takeout, or eat food that's prepared anywhere but in your own kitchen.

How Portion Sizes Have Changed		
Food Item	**Calories per Portion Twenty Years Ago**	**Calories per Portion Today**
Bagel	140 calories (3-inch diameter)	360 calories (4-inch diameter)
Fast-food cheeseburger	333 calories	590 calories
Spaghetti and meatballs	500 calories (1 cup of spaghetti with sauce and 3 small meatballs)	1,025 calories (2 cups of spaghetti and 3 large meatballs)
Bottle of soda	85 calories (6.5 ounces)	250 calories (20 ounces)
Fast-food French fries	210 calories (2.4 ounces)	610 calories (6.9 ounces)
Turkey sandwich	320 calories	820 calories (10-inch sub)

Source: Adapted from the Portion Distortion Quiz on the Heart, Lung, and Blood Institute Web site.

PART TWO

What You *Can* Eat: Easy Menus and Mouth-Watering Recipes

7

Your Meal Plan

This chapter contains two weeks of menu plans that are consistent with the Dietary Guidelines recommendations. On average, they provide approximately 2,000 calories (see chapter 2 to determine the daily meal plan that's right for your calorie level). After I created these menus, I used a computerized nutritional analysis program to make certain not only that they followed the daily meal plan for a 2,000-calorie diet, but that on average they met the guidelines' daily recommendations for total fat (20 to 35 percent of total calories), saturated fat (less than 10 percent of total calories), dietary choles-terol (less than 300 mg), and sodium (less than 2,300 mg), and were low in trans fats and added sugars as well. On each day you will see asterisked (*) items; these indicate recipes that, along with twenty others, can be found in chapter 8.

Each food item in the menus, as well as each recipe, has a break-down for the approximate amount of food from each food category to assist you in planning your meals or to enable you to substitute other choices within those respective food groups. See chapter 3, as well as appendix A, for more food and meal ideas.

If your daily meal plan is for 2,000 calories, you can follow this menu plan as is. If your calorie needs are more or less, find the appropriate meal plan to meet your needs and either reduce or increase your portions accordingly (see chapter 2 for "Suggested

Daily Amount of Food from Each Food Group"). To adapt the menu to provide about 1,600 calories, you could subtract ½ cup fruit, ½ cup vegetables, a 1-ounce equivalent of grains, a ½-ounce equivalent of meat and beans, 1 teaspoon of oil, and 135 discretionary calories. Someone who requires about 2,600 calories can add 1 cup of vegetables, three extra 1-ounce servings of grains (preferably some whole grains), a 1-ounce equivalent of meat and beans, 1 teaspoon of oil, and 143 discretionary calories.

Day 1

BREAKFAST

1 cup cooked oatmeal (2 whole grains)
1 teaspoon trans fat–free margarine (1 oil)
1 cup sliced strawberries (1 cup fruit)
1 cup skim milk (1 milk)

LUNCH

Tuna salad sandwich:
  3 ounces light tuna, packed in water (3 meats and beans)
  2 tablespoons light mayonnaise (2 oils)
  2 leaves romaine lettuce (¼ cup vegetables)
  2 slices tomato (¼ cup vegetables)
  1 large whole-wheat pita, 2 ounces (2 whole grains)
1 cup baby carrots (1 cup vegetables)
1 cup skim milk (1 milk)

DINNER

Chicken and Broccoli Pasta* (1⅛ cups vegetables, 2 grains, 5 meats and beans, 2¼ oils, plus 44 discretionary calories)
5 ounces red wine (115 discretionary calories)
1 large orange (1 cup fruit)

SNACKS/DESSERTS

8 ounces plain low-fat yogurt (1 milk plus 110 discretionary calories), topped with ¼ cup low-fat granola (1 whole grain) and a sprinkle of cinnamon
1 cup blueberries (1 cup fruit)

Day 2

BREAKFAST

1½ cups oat bran flakes (1½ whole grains)

1 cup skim milk (1 milk)

1 cup grapefruit sections (1 cup fruit)

LUNCH

3 oz. grilled chicken breast, skinless, boneless, cut into strips
(3 meats and beans)

2 cups romaine lettuce (1 cup vegetables)

¼ cup chopped walnuts (1 meat and beans)

½ cup red grapes, sliced in half (½ cup fruit)

½ cup chopped green apple (½ cup fruit)

½ cup cherry tomatoes (½ cup vegetables)

2 tablespoons Creamy Buttermilk Dressing* (1½ oils)

1 whole-grain roll, 2 ounces (2 whole grains)

1 teaspoon trans fat–free margarine (1 oil)

DINNER

3 ounces grilled flank steak (3 meats and beans)

1 cup roasted red potatoes* (1¾ cups vegetables plus
2 oils)

1 cup steamed asparagus (1 cup vegetables)

1 teaspoon trans fat–free margarine (1 oil)

SNACKS/DESSERTS

1 cup low-fat lemon yogurt (1 milk plus 110 discretionary
calories), mixed with 1 cup raspberries (1 cup fruit)

Cheese and crackers: 10 saltine crackers (1½ grains), topped
with 1½ ounces low-fat cheddar cheese (1 milk)

2 graham cracker squares (2 grams)

Day 3

BREAKFAST

2 whole-wheat waffles (2 whole grains)

2 teaspoons trans fat–free margarine (2 oils)

1 cup raspberries (1 cup fruit)

1 cup skim milk (1 milk)

LUNCH

Turkey and Cheese Pinwheels:

> 3 ounces fresh roasted turkey (3 meats and beans)
>
> 2 ounces low-fat Swiss cheese (1 milk plus 28 discretionary calories)
>
> 2 leaves romaine lettuce (¼ cup vegetables)
>
> 2 slices tomato (¼ cup vegetables)
>
> 1 tablespoon mustard
>
> 1 tablespoon light mayonnaise (1 oil)
>
> 1 large whole-wheat flour tortilla, 2 ounces (2 whole grains)

1 cup baby carrots (1 cup vegetables)

DINNER

4 ounces Baked Cod Fish* (4 meats plus ¼ grain)

2 cups spinach salad (1 cup vegetables) with 2 tablespoons Garlic Lemon Vinaigrette* (3 oils)

1 cup wild rice (2 whole grains)

SNACKS/DESSERTS

1 cup low-fat vanilla yogurt (1 milk plus 110 discretionary calories), topped with a sprinkle of cinnamon

1 cup fat-free chocolate fudge pudding (100 discretionary calories)

2 large plums (1 cup fruit)

Day 4

BREAKFAST

Cheesy Vegetable Omelet* (½ cup vegetables, 1½ meats and beans plus 1 milk)

1 slice whole-wheat toast (1 whole grain)

1 teaspoon trans fat–free margarine (1 oil)

1 cup orange juice (1 cup fruit)

LUNCH

Corny Bean Salad* (½ cup vegetables, 2 lean meats and beans plus 3 oils)

1 cup skim milk (1 milk)

DINNER

Chicken Quesadilla* (¾ cup vegetables, 2 whole grains, 4 meats and beans, ¼ milk, 1½ oils)

½ cup Spanish rice (1 grain)

SNACKS/DESSERTS

1 cup nonfat plain yogurt (1 milk), topped with 2 tablespoons chopped cashews (1 meat and beans plus 1 oil) and 2 tablespoons dried cranberries (½ cup fruit)

½ cup vanilla ice cream (½ milk plus 100 discretionary calories), topped with ½ cup blueberries (½ cup fruit)

1 cup raw vegetables (1 cup vegetables)

Day 5

BREAKFAST

Combined in a bowl: ½ cup low-fat cottage cheese (1 milk), 1 cup cantaloupe balls (1 cup fruit), and 1 ounce shaved almonds (2 lean meat and beans plus 2 oils)

1 slice whole-wheat toast (1 whole grain)

1 teaspoon trans fat–free margarine (1 oil)

LUNCH

Crunchy Egg Salad* (1½ lean meats and beans, 2 oils)

1 cup sliced fresh peaches (1 cup fruit)

1 cup skim milk (1 milk)

DINNER

Bean burrito:

½ cup black beans, canned, drained (2 meats and beans)

1 large whole-wheat burrito (2 whole grains)

1 slice American cheese (½ milk plus 40 discretionary calories)

1½ cups broccoli (1½ cups vegetables), sautéed in 2 teaspoons olive oil (2 oils)

SNACKS/DESSERTS

Mango-Banana Smoothie* (1 cup fruit, ½ milk plus 20 discretionary calories)

2 graham cracker squares (1 grain), topped with 2 tablespoons natural peanut butter (2 meats and beans plus 2 oils)

1 cup sliced cucumbers and cherry tomatoes (1 cup vegetables), dipped in 1 tablespoon Italian dressing (1 oil)

Tall mocha latte made with nonfat milk (1 milk plus 30 discretionary calories)

Day 6

BREAKFAST

1 whole-wheat English muffin (2 whole grains)

2 teaspoons almond butter (2 meats and beans plus 2 oils)

1 cup low-fat plain yogurt (1 milk plus 110 discretionary calories)

1 cup blueberries (1 cup fruit)

LUNCH

Vegetable Mozzarella Pizza* (1 cup vegetables, 2 whole grains, 1 milk, 3 oils plus 60 discretionary calories)

1 cup skim milk (1 milk)

DINNER

Linda's Chicken Meatballs and Spaghetti* (½ cup vegetables, 2 grains, 4 meats and beans plus 25 discretionary calories)

Chopped salad:

2 cups romaine lettuce, chopped (1 cup vegetables)

½ cup chopped yellow tomato (½ cup vegetables)

½ cup shredded carrots (½ cup vegetables)

2 tablespoons ranch dressing, reduced-fat (2 oils)

SNACKS/DESSERTS

2 tablespoons (½ ounce) unsalted shaved almonds (1 meat and beans plus 1 oil), mixed with ¼ cup raisins (½ cup fruit)

3 pretzel rods (1 grain)

½ cup strawberry frozen yogurt (½ milk plus 70 discretionary calories)

½ cup green grapes (½ cup fruit)

Day 7

BREAKFAST

Bacon Vegetable Scramble* (½ cup vegetables, 1½ meats and beans, 1 milk)

1 whole-wheat English muffin, toasted (2 whole grains)

2 teaspoons trans fat–free margarine (2 oils)

½ pink grapefruit (½ cup fruit)

1 cup skim milk (1 milk)

LUNCH

Roasted turkey sandwich:

3 slices fresh white meat turkey, roasted (3 meats and beans)

Apple Coleslaw* (1 cup vegetables, ½ oil plus 10 discretionary calories)

2 slices whole-wheat bread, toasted (2 whole grains)

1 cup orange juice (1 cup fruit)

DINNER

Olive and Sun-Dried Tomato Pasta* (½ cup vegetables, 2 grains, 2½ oils)

SNACKS/DESSERTS

1 cup low-fat vanilla yogurt (1 milk plus 110 discretionary calories), topped with ¼ cup dried apricots (½ cup fruit)

1 ounce cashews (2 meats and beans plus 2 oils)

1 large banana (1 cup fruit)

1 ounce jelly beans (106 discretionary calories)
½ cup baby carrots (½ cup vegetables)

Day 8

BREAKFAST

Sweetest Potato Pancakes* (2 grains, ½ cup vegetables)
1 teaspoon trans fat–free margarine (1 oil)
1 teaspoon light maple syrup (8 discretionary calories)
1 banana (½ cup fruit)
1 cup skim milk (1 milk)

LUNCH

1 vegetable burger (2 meats and beans)
1 whole-wheat hamburger bun (2 whole grains)
2 leaves romaine lettuce (¼ cup vegetables)
2 slices tomato (¼ cup vegetables)
1 slice reduced-fat American cheese, melted (⅓ milk)
1 tablespoon ketchup (15 discretionary calories)
1 cup seedless red grapes (1 cup fruit)

DINNER

Lemon Garlic Chicken* (4 lean meats and beans plus 1½ oils)
½ cup brown rice (1 whole grain)
1 teaspoon trans fat–free margarine (1 oil)
1 cup cauliflower (1 cup vegetables) and ½ cup carrots (½ cup vegetables), sautéed in 2 teaspoons olive oil (2 oils)

SNACKS/DESSERTS

½ cup vanilla ice cream (½ milk plus 100 discretionary calories), topped with 1 tablespoon chocolate syrup (20 discretionary calories)
5 whole grain crackers (1 whole grain), topped with 1 tablespoon natural peanut butter (1 meat and beans plus 1 oil)
1 cup low-fat vanilla yogurt (1 milk plus 110 discretionary calories), topped with ½ cup fresh sliced strawberries (½ cup fruit)

Day 9

BREAKFAST

Cheesy Cinnamon Raisin Toast* (1 cup fruit, 2 whole grains, 2 oils plus 1 milk)

1 cup fresh pineapple chunks (1 cup fruit)

LUNCH

Salad made with:

1 cup bibb lettuce ($\frac{1}{2}$ cup vegetables)

1 cup red leaf lettuce ($\frac{1}{2}$ cup vegetables)

$\frac{1}{2}$ cup yellow tomato ($\frac{1}{2}$ cup vegetables)

1 ounce chopped walnuts (2 meats and beans plus 2 oils)

1 pear, chopped ($\frac{1}{2}$ cup fruit)

$1\frac{1}{2}$ ounces fresh mozzarella cheese (1 milk plus 45 discretionary calories)

1 hard-boiled egg (1 meat and beans)

3 ounces grilled chicken breast (3 meats and beans)

$\frac{1}{2}$ cup croutons (1 grain)

2 tablespoons Italian salad dressing (2 oils)

DINNER

1 cup penne (2 grains), topped with 2 cups Vegetable and Bean Tomato Sauce* (2 cups vegetables, 2 meats and beans plus $1\frac{1}{2}$ oils)

SNACKS/DESSERTS

1 large fresh peach (1 cup fruit)

1 cup nonfat yogurt (1 milk), topped with $\frac{1}{4}$ cup Grape Nuts cereal (1 whole grain) plus 1 ounce unsalted peanuts (2 meats and beans plus 2 oils)

Day 10

BREAKFAST

1 cup oatmeal (2 whole grains)

1 teaspoon trans fat–free margarine (1 oil)

½ teaspoon brown sugar (8 discretionary calories)

2 tablespoons walnuts, chopped (1 meat and beans plus 1 oil)

1 small orange, sliced (½ cup fruit)

1 cup skim milk (1 cup milk)

LUNCH

Fabulous Feta Chicken Salad Sandwich* (1 cup vegetables, 2 whole grains, 2 meats and beans, 1 milk, 3 oils)

1 cup honeydew, cubed (1 cup fruit)

DINNER

Sensational Salmon* (½ cup vegetables, 4 lean meats and beans, 20 discretionary calories)

Garlic Brussels Sprouts* (1¼ cups vegetables, 3 oils)

1 cup couscous (2 grains) made with 1 teaspoon olive oil (1 oil)

5 ounces red wine (115 discretionary calories)

SNACKS/DESSERTS

2 Oatmeal Applesauce Cookies* (120 discretionary calories)

1 cup sweet fresh cherries (1 cup fruit)

1 cup skim milk (1 milk)

Day 11

BREAKFAST

Peppy Pumpkin Muffins* (1 whole-grain, ¼ cup fruit plus 1 oil)

1 cup nonfat vanilla yogurt (1 milk)

2 tablespoons walnuts, chopped (1 meat and beans plus 1 oil)

½ grapefruit (½ cup fruit)

LUNCH

Tasty Tuna Ties* (½ cup vegetables, 2 grains, 3 meats and beans plus 2 oils)

1 cup watermelon balls (1 cup fruit)

1 cup skim milk (1 milk)

DINNER

Tofu Teriyaki Stir-Fry* (2 cups vegetables, 2 meats and beans,
3 oils plus 8 discretionary calories)

1 cup brown rice (2 whole grains)

SNACKS/DESSERTS

1 cup frozen yogurt (1 milk plus 140 discretionary calories),
topped with ½ cup blackberries (½ cup fruit)

2 small chocolate chip cookies (100 discretionary calories)

Day 12

BREAKFAST

1 slice whole-wheat toast (1 whole grain)

1 teaspoon apple butter (10 discretionary calories)

yogurt parfait made with ½ cup kiwi (½ cup fruit) and ½ cup
mango (½ cup fruit), 1 cup nonfat plain yogurt (1 milk), and
¼ cup low-fat granola (1 whole grain)

LUNCH

Gemelli Chicken Caesar Salad* (⅝ cup vegetables, 2 grains,
3 meats and beans, ½ milk, 2 oils, 15 discretionary calories)

1 cup skim milk (1 milk)

DINNER

Nana Burgers* (¼ cup vegetables, 4 meats and beans, 1 oil)

1 whole-wheat hamburger bun (2 whole grains)

1 cup spaghetti squash (1 cup vegetables) served with ½ cup
tomato sauce (½ cup vegetables) and 2 tablespoons grated
cheese (40 discretionary calories)

SNACKS/DESSERTS

1 large apple (1 cup fruit)

1 almond biscotti (120 discretionary calories)

1 cup skim milk (1 milk)

Day 13

BREAKFAST

1 cup MultiGrain Cheerios (1 whole grain)

1 cup sliced strawberries (1 cup fruit)

1 cup skim milk (1 milk)

LUNCH

Burrito made with:

Molly's Marvelous Lentils* (1½ cups vegetables, 1 meat and beans plus ½ oil)

1 7- or 8-inch flour tortilla (2 grains)

¼ cup low-fat shredded cheddar cheese (½ milk)

1 cup romaine lettuce (½ cup vegetables)

2 tablespoons creamy ranch dressing (2 oils)

1 cup skim milk (1 milk)

DINNER

3-ounce pork chop, grilled (3 meats and beans)

Asparagus and Mushrooms with Fresh Coriander* (1¼ cups vegetables)

1 cup brown rice (2 whole grains)

1 teaspoon trans fat–free margarine (1 oil)

5 ounces white wine (115 discretionary calories)

SNACKS/DESSERTS

1 ounce whole-wheat pretzels (1 whole grain)

½ cup low-fat yogurt (½ milk plus 50 discretionary calories) mixed with ½ cup raspberries (½ cup fruit)

¼ cup raisins (½ cup fruit), mixed with 2 tablespoons (½ ounce) unsalted, dry-roasted peanuts (1 meat and beans plus 1 oil)

Day 14

BREAKFAST

1 whole-wheat English muffin (2 whole grains), toasted,
 topped with 1 tablespoon low-fat whipped cream cheese
 (35 discretionary calories) and ½ cup sliced apricots
 (½ cup fruit)

1 cup skim milk (1 cup milk)

LUNCH

2 slices deli turkey breast, oven roasted (2 meats and beans)

1 slice Swiss cheese, reduced-sodium (⅔ milk plus 40 discretionary calories)

1 teaspoon mustard

1 teaspoon light mayonnaise (1 oil)

1 hoagie roll (2 grains)

½ cup baby carrots (½ cup vegetables)

1 cup mixed fruit salad (1 cup fruit)

1 cup skim milk (1 milk)

DINNER

Crunchy Chicken Nuggets* (4 meats and beans, ½ grain)

1 russet potato, baked (1 cup vegetables), topped with 1
 teaspoon trans fat–free margarine (1 oil)

1 cup green beans (1 cup vegetables), sautéed in 2 teaspoons
 olive oil (2 oils) and topped with 2 tablespoons (½ ounce)
 shaved almonds (1 meat and beans plus 1 oil)

SNACKS/DESSERTS

1 cup nonfat plain yogurt (1 milk), topped with ½ cup
 mandarin orange slices (½ cup fruit)

4 cups unsalted popcorn (1½ whole grains), topped with 2
 teaspoons canola oil (2 oils)

1 large banana (1 cup fruit)

8

Recipes

The following recipes, using many healthful and delicious ingredients, can easily be incorporated into your individualized meal plan. Keep in mind that many of these recipes would work well for different meals throughout the day, so feel free to have Sweetest Potato Pancakes, typically a breakfast dish, as a side dish for dinner, or enjoy Penne with Olives and Sausage as a cold pasta salad for lunch instead of having it as a warm dish at dinner. Also, feel free to reduce the amount you consume of any recipe if you want to include it but feel the recommended serving sizes are too large.

Breakfasts

Cheesy Vegetable Omelet

This is one of my husband's favorite weekend recipes—it's simple, takes only a few minutes to prepare, and packs a powerful protein punch to give us an energy boost for the day. It also gives us a head start on meeting our daily vegetable quota.

nonstick cooking spray
2 large egg whites, raw
1 egg yolk, raw
¼ cup red onion, chopped
¼ cup fresh tomato, chopped
1 teaspoon chives
1 ounce low-fat Swiss cheese

Total preparation and cooking time: 15 minutes

Makes 1 serving.

Nutrition information per serving:
Calories: 170
Fat: 6 g
  Saturated fat: 2.5 g
  Monounsaturated fat: 0 g
Cholesterol: 210 mg
Sodium: 90 mg
Carbohydrate: 10 g
Fiber: 1 g
Protein: 17 g

On medium heat, coat the bottom of a nonstick medium frying pan with nonstick cooking spray. Mix the egg whites and egg yolk in a bowl, and when the frying pan is hot, add the eggs to the pan and let them set for 1 minute. Slide the pan gently and bring the eggs to the center. Add the onion, tomato, chives, and Swiss cheese to one side of the eggs. After 1 minute, gently fold the egg to make an omelet.

Cook's tip: You can replace the onion, tomato, or chives with mushrooms, peppers, or other vegetables as desired. You can also substitute cheddar, American, or any other cheese you prefer instead of Swiss or omit it entirely. If you scramble the eggs, you can serve more people.

Bacon Vegetable Scramble

The addition of just one slice of Canadian bacon adds great flavor and texture to scrambled eggs.

- 2 large egg whites, raw
- ¼ cup red peppers, chopped
- ¼ cup yellow peppers, chopped
- 2 ounces low-fat cheddar cheese, shredded
- 1 slice of Canadian bacon, chopped

Coat the bottom of a nonstick medium frying pan and set it on medium heat. When hot, pour the egg whites in the pan. Add the red and yellow peppers, cheddar cheese, and bacon, and stir gently to combine the ingredients. When cooked, remove from heat and serve immediately.

Cook's TIP: This tastes great on a toasted whole-wheat English muffin.

Total preparation and cooking time: 15 minutes

Makes 1 serving.

Nutrition information per serving:

Calories: 200
Fat: 6 g
  Saturated fat: 3 g
  Monounsaturated fat: 3 g
Cholesterol: 25 mg
Sodium: 820 mg
Carbohydrate: 6 g
Fiber: 1 g
Protein: 27 g

Randi's Mushroom Frittata

This dish is a real winner. My family and I were lucky enough to enjoy our friend Randi's delicious recipe for brunch not long ago.

- 12-inch nonstick pan that can go from stovetop to oven
- 2 teaspoons olive oil
- 6 large eggs
- 4 egg whites
- 1 cup 1% milk (it's better if not skim)
- salt and pepper to taste
- 12 mushrooms sliced thin
- 4 ounces smoked gouda cheese, shredded
- 6 leaves fresh basil, finely chopped

Total preparation and cooking time: 20 to 30 minutes

Makes 6 servings.

Nutrition information per serving: (includes ⅛ teaspoon salt)

Calories: 190
Fat: 12 g
  Saturated fat: 5 g
  Monounsaturated fat: 5 g
Cholesterol: 235 mg
Sodium: 330 mg
Carbohydrate: 4 g
Fiber: 0 g
Protein: 16 g

Preheat the broiler on high. Set the skillet with the olive oil on medium heat. In a large bowl whisk together the eggs, egg whites, and milk with salt and pepper. Add the mushrooms to the skillet, and cook them for about 5 minutes until lightly browned. Over medium heat, add the egg mixture to the skillet with the mushrooms. Mix them together, and then add the cheese and basil. Gently lift the eggs at the sides and let the uncooked eggs move around so that the eggs cook slowly and evenly (as if you are making an omelet—not scrambled eggs). When the eggs are mostly cooked throughout (after about 10 minutes), put the entire skillet in the broiler (about 6 inches under the flame) for 1 to 3 minutes until the top is fluffy and golden. Remove it from the oven, and serve it in wedges.

Cook's tip: Randi uses a 12-inch nonstick pan so that the frittata is thin and stays fluffy, and she likes to use fresh herbs. Another delicious combination she loves to make is asparagus, goat cheese, and tarragon.

Sweetest Potato Pancakes

Adding sweet potatoes to pancakes is a great way to incorporate more vegetables (and more vitamin A, as well as fiber) into your day. They are easy to prepare and can help your kids (who may shy away from vegetables) meet their daily vegetable quota.

1 medium sweet potato
nonstick cooking spray
⅔ cup pancake and waffle mix, complete, dry
⅛ teaspoon cinnamon
¾ cup water
2 teaspoons powdered sugar

Total preparation and cooking time: 15–20 minutes

Makes 2 servings.

Nutrition information per serving:
Calories: 230
Fat: 3 g
  Saturated fat: 0.5 g
  Monounsaturated fat: 2.5 g
Cholesterol: 10 mg
Sodium: 520 mg
Carbohydrate: 47 g
Fiber: 3 g
Protein: 6 g

Clean the sweet potato, poke it with a fork, wrap it in a paper towel, and microwave it for 7 or 8 minutes or until you can easily put a fork in it. Set it aside. Spray a griddle or a large pan with the cooking spray, and set it on medium heat. Pour the pancake and waffle mix into a large bowl, along with the cinnamon, and add water to the mix (add more water for fluffier pancakes, less for denser pancakes). Scoop out the sweet potato and add it to the mix. Combine the ingredients until the desired texture is achieved. Cook the pancakes on a griddle or in a large pan (you can make 2 large pancakes or 4 smaller ones). Watch the pancakes carefully, and flip them after 3 or 4 minutes or until they're solid. Cook them another 3 or 4 minutes, and remove them from the heat promptly. Sprinkle on powdered sugar and serve.

Cook's tip: You can replace the sweet potato with applesauce, a ripe banana, or blueberries; it's a great way to sneak some fruit into your day. You can make more pancakes to freeze, and pop them in the microwave oven for a quick and easy breakfast, dessert, or even dinner side dish.

Cheesy Cinnamon Raisin Toast

My mother declares that this simple, easy-to-make breakfast or midday snack "tastes like a cheese Danish." She has satisfied her sweet tooth with this fiber- and protein-rich meal for years.

2 slices whole-wheat bread, toasted
2 teaspoons trans fat–free margarine
½ cup low-fat, low-sodium cottage cheese
¼ cup golden seedless raisins
½ teaspoon cinnamon, ground

Toast the whole-wheat bread. Top it with the margarine. Then add the cottage cheese and raisins, and sprinkle with cinnamon. Heat it for 3 minutes in a toaster oven and serve.

Cook's tip: This can make a great breakfast or an in-between meal snack.

Total preparation and cooking time: 5 minutes

Makes 1 serving.

Nutrition information per serving:
Calories: 400
Fat: 11 g
   Saturated fat: 2.5 g
   Monounsaturated fat: 5 g
Cholesterol: 5 mg
Sodium: 417 mg
Carbohydrate: 59 g
Fiber: 6 g
Protein: 21 g

Peppy Pumpkin Muffins

These muffins are a great way to get pumpkin, rich in vitamin A, into your diet. They make a great on-the-go breakfast with a cup of skim milk or a delicious anytime snack.

1½ cups whole-wheat flour
1 cup unbleached flour
¾ cups sugar
2 tablespoons baking powder
2 teaspoons ground cinnamon
½ teaspoon ground nutmeg
¼ teaspoon salt
6 egg whites, slightly beaten
1 cup skim milk
½ cup canola oil
1 tablespoon vanilla
1 cup canned pumpkin
¾ cup raisins, chopped

Total preparation and cooking time: 45 minutes

Makes 21 servings.

Nutrition information per serving:
Calories: 140
Fat: 6 g
  Saturated fat: 0 g
  Monounsaturated fat: 5 g
Cholesterol: 0 mg
Sodium: 190 mg
Carbohydrate: 22 g
Fiber: 2 g
Protein: 3 g

Preheat the oven to 350 degrees F. Place 21 paper baking cups in muffin tins. In a very large bowl, mix the flour, sugar, baking powder, cinnamon, nutmeg, and salt thoroughly, and set them aside. In a separate bowl, mix the egg whites, skim milk, canola oil, and vanilla. Add this to the flour mixture. Then add the pumpkin and raisins, and stir until the dry ingredients are barely moistened. Fill each paper cup two-thirds full. Bake for 20 minutes or until a toothpick inserted in the center comes out clean. Remove the muffins from the tins and cool.

Cook's tip: You can freeze these and pop them in a toaster oven to heat and eat in a hurry. Add some low-fat yogurt or skim milk and voilà—you have a meal!

Salads and Soups

Corny Bean Salad

This flavorful salad is also very filling, as it contains fiber-rich beans, corn, and other vegetables.

½ cup kidney beans, canned and drained
½ cup fresh sweet corn kernels
1 tablespoon red wine vinegar
1 tablespoon extra-virgin olive oil
½ teaspoon cumin seeds, ground
1 tablespoon fresh parsley
1 scallion, chopped

In a large bowl, combine the kidney beans, corn, red wine vinegar, olive oil, cumin seeds, parsley, and scallions. Toss, chill (if desired), and serve.

COOK'S TIP: You can substitute chickpeas or another favorite bean for the beans in this salad and can add other vegetables as desired.

Total preparation and cooking time: 10 minutes

Makes 1 serving.

Nutrition information per serving:
Calories: 305
Fat: 16 g
  Saturated fat: 2 g
  Monounsaturated fat: 11 g
Cholesterol: 0 mg
Sodium: 400 mg
Carbohydrate: 35 g
Fiber: 8 g
Protein: 10 g

Crunchy Egg Salad

My mom's famous recipe tastes great straight from the refrigerator! It gives you the taste and texture of traditional egg salad, with less fat and fewer calories.

3 large eggs, raw (2 yolks will not be used)
1 5-inch celery stalk, chopped
1 scallion, chopped
2 tablespoons light mayonnaise
1 teaspoon mustard
½ teaspoon paprika

Total preparation and cooking time: 15 minutes

Makes 1 serving.

Nutrition information per serving:
Calories: 215
Fat: 15 g
  Saturated fat: 1.5 g
  Monounsaturated fat: 7.0 g
Cholesterol: 215 mg
Sodium: 491 mg
Carbohydrate: 7.5 g
Fiber: 1 g
Protein: 14 g

In a pan, cover the eggs in cold water. Set the pan on high heat. When the water boils, lower the heat to a simmer. Cover for 5 minutes. Turn off the heat and let the eggs sit for 5 minutes. Once they're cooked, run cold water over them to seize the shells (and make them easy to peel). Carefully peel the shells. Discard two yolks, and place the remaining eggs (3 whites with 1 yolk) into a bowl. Mash with a fork. Add the celery, scallion, mayonnaise, mustard, and paprika, and combine the ingredients until creamy. Chill and serve.

Cook's tip: Serve this on toasted bread with lettuce and tomato or on crispy crackers or rice cakes. It also tastes great over salad greens.

Gemelli Chicken Caesar Salad

My caterer, Alicia Reinish, the owner of Catered Word, first introduced me to the idea of mixing pasta with chicken Caesar salad. This is a hearty and satisfying meal that pleases your taste buds with its unique combination of ingredients.

2 tablespoons light Caesar salad dressing
1 tablespoon light mayonnaise
⅛ teaspoon pepper
3 ounces grilled chicken breast, cut into cubes or strips
1 cup romaine lettuce
½ cup croutons
½ ounce pine nuts (about 2 tablespoons), toasted
2 sun-dried tomatoes
2 tablespoons grated parmesan cheese
2 ounces gemelli pasta (⅔ cup dry), cooked and drained

Total preparation and cooking time: 20–25 minutes

Makes 1 serving.

Nutrition information per serving:

Calories: 600
Fat: 22 g
 Saturated fat: 5 g
 Monounsaturated fat: 7.5 g
Cholesterol: 65 mg
Sodium: 860 mg
Carbohydrate: 66 g
Fiber: 5 g
Protein: 37 g

In a serving bowl, combine the Caesar salad dressing, mayonnaise, and pepper. Add the chicken, romaine, croutons, pine nuts, tomatoes, parmesan cheese, and pasta. Toss until evenly coated. Cover, chill, and serve.

COOK'S TIP: You can replace the gemelli with a more familiar pasta like penne, but the gemelli does add a firm yet appealing texture to the salad.

Veggie Taco Salad

This recipe, courtesy of my friend Cynthia, provides a great balance of protein, carbohydrates, and healthful fat. It is filling and delicious.

⅓ ripe avocado
¼ cup soy crumbles (Boca Burger or Morningstar Farms)
½ cup vegetarian refried beans (canned)
2 cups torn romaine leaves
¼ cup tomatoes, chopped
¼ cup onions, chopped
5 blue corn tortilla chips, crumbled

Total preparation and cooking time: 15 minutes

Makes 1 serving.

Nutrition information per serving:
Calories: 480
Fat: 23 g
    Saturated fat: 2 g
    Monounsaturated fat: 7 g
Cholesterol: 0 mg
Sodium: 1430 mg
Carbohydrate: 52 g
Fiber: 18 g
Protein: 21 g

Mash the avocado, then chill. Heat the soy crumbles in a microwave for 45 seconds. Set them aside. Heat the beans in the microwave for 30 to 40 seconds. Place the romaine in a salad bowl. Toss in the avocado, beans, soy crumbles, tomatoes, and onions. Sprinkle crumbled tortilla chips on top of the bean mixture.

COOK'S TIP: This is a great and flavorful dish but is high in sodium. To lower the sodium content, you can buy lower-sodium ingredients (such as low-sodium beans) or, better yet, have a half portion and enjoy the full flavor of this dish!

Warm Mediterranean Spinach Salad

This salad is a lively way to include vegetables in a meal. The small amount of crumbled bacon, while high in saturated fat and sodium, adds great flavor.

4 cups baby spinach, washed, cold
3 tablespoons extra-virgin olive oil
6 ounces portobello mushrooms, sliced
   length-wise
8 cloves garlic, diced
½ teaspoon balsamic vinegar
½ teaspoon Dijon mustard
½ cup reduced-calorie bacon bits
pepper to taste

Total preparation and cooking time: 15–20 minutes

Makes 4 servings.

Nutrition information per serving:

Calories: 140
Fat: 10 g
   Saturated fat: 2 g
   Monounsaturated fat: 8 g
Cholesterol: 10 mg
Sodium: 530 mg
Carbohydrate: 7 g
Fiber: 2 g
Protein: 7 g

Place the spinach in a bowl in the refrigerator. Heat the oil in a large nonstick skillet. Wipe the portobello mushrooms with a damp paper towel to remove the extra dirt. Sauté the mushrooms in the oil until they're soft. Add the garlic, vinegar, and mustard. Cook for 1 minute. Add the bacon bits and pepper. Serve over cold spinach leaves.

Cook's TIP: Top this salad with sliced grilled chicken to make it a main course.

Creamy Buttermilk Dressing

My mom created this dressing as an alternative to commercial salad dressings, which are often loaded with fat and sodium.

2 tablespoons light mayonnaise
3 tablespoons buttermilk, low-fat
1/4 teaspoon garlic powder or 1 small garlic
  clove, finely chopped
2 teaspoons fresh lemon juice
1/2 teaspoon parsley, finely chopped
1/2 teaspoon East Indian yellow curry powder
1/4 teaspoon salt

Total preparation and cooking time: 10 minutes

Makes 2 servings.

Nutrition information per serving:
Calories: 60
Fat: 5 g
  Saturated fat: 1g
  Monounsaturated fat: 0 g
Cholesterol: 5 mg
Sodium: 440 mg
Carbohydrate: 3 g
Fiber: 0 g
Protein: 1 g

In a small bowl, combine the mayonnaise, buttermilk, garlic powder, lemon juice, parsley, curry powder, and salt. Refrigerate until serving.

Cook's TIP: This can be used to top salad greens but also works well in place of sour cream on a baked Idaho potato or a sweet potato. This dressing can add color and flavor to a poached fish or chicken dish.

Garlic Lemon Vinaigrette

This is my mom's own recipe, which adds a nice blend of tartness and smoothness to a salad.

4 tablespoons extra-virgin olive oil
1 tablespoon fresh lemon juice
1 garlic clove, finely chopped
1½ tablespoons balsamic vinegar
1 tablespoon fresh dill, finely chopped
1 tablespoon fresh parsley, finely chopped
¼ teaspoon salt
pinch of pepper

In a small bowl combine the olive oil, lemon juice, garlic, vinegar, dill, parsley, salt, and pepper. Chill and serve.

COOK'S TIP: This dressing can be used not only to top spinach, romaine, or other lettuce leaves, but also as a dip for fresh cut-up carrots, cherry tomatoes, or sliced cucumbers.

Total preparation and cooking time: 15 minutes

Makes 4 servings.

Nutrition information per serving:
Calories: 140
Fat: 14 g
  Saturated fat: 2 g
  Monounsaturated fat: 12 g
Cholesterol: 0 mg
Sodium: 150 mg
Carbohydrate: 2 g
Fiber: 0 g
Protein: 0 g

Spinach Orange Salad

This recipe pairs fruits with vegetables to create a low-calorie salad packed with fiber and vitamins A and C. The light orange juice dressing adds a sweet-tart flavor.

4 cups spinach, washed and torn into pieces
2 medium oranges, sectioned
zest from 1 orange, grated
½ cup red onion, sliced
⅔ cup mushrooms, sliced
¼ cup orange juice
1 tablespoon vinegar
½ teaspoon vegetable oil
½ teaspoon ground ginger
¼ teaspoon pepper

Total preparation and cooking time: 20 minutes

Makes 4 servings.

Nutrition information per serving:
Calories: 70
Fat: 1 g
  Saturated fat: 0 g
  Monounsaturated fat: 0 g
Cholesterol: 0 mg
Sodium: 25 mg
Carbohydrate: 16 g
Fiber: 5 g
Protein: 2 g

Place the spinach in a bowl. Add the orange sections and the zest, onion, and mushrooms. Toss them lightly to mix. Mix the orange juice, vinegar, oil, ginger, and pepper well. Pour this over the spinach mixture. Toss and chill.

COOK'S TIP: This salad tastes great with a baked skinless chicken breast, seasoned lima beans, and a hot, crispy whole-grain roll.

Broccoli Onion Soup

This soup is a great way to get in some vegetables and key nutrients like vitamin C, but it's also a tasty starter for a meal. Unlike some soups, this one is low in sodium and can fill you up with few calories.

Total preparation and cooking time: 20 minutes

Makes 4 servings.

Nutrition information per serving:
Calories: 45
Fat: 2 g
  Saturated fat: 1.5 g
  Monounsaturated fat: 0 g
Cholesterol: 10 mg
Sodium: 60 mg
Carbohydrate: 4 g
Fiber: 1 g
Protein: 4 g

2 cups broccoli, chopped
¼ cup celery, diced
¼ cup onion, chopped
1 cup chicken broth, unsalted
2 tablespoons skim milk
salt to taste
pepper to taste
thyme, ground to taste
¼ cup Swiss cheese, shredded

Put the vegetables and the chicken broth in a saucepan. Bring this to a boil, reduce the heat, cover, and cook until the vegetables are tender—about 8 minutes. Mix the milk, salt, pepper, and thyme; add this to the cooked vegetables. Cook, stirring constantly, until the soup is slightly thickened and the mixture just begins to boil. Remove it from the heat. Add the cheese and stir until it's melted.

Cook's tip: You can use more colorful vegetables like carrots in this recipe to add vitamin A and other key nutrients, while still
keeping calories and sodium down.

Audree's Famous Chicken Soup

*This recipe is from the late mother and the
mother-in-law, respectively, of our dear
friends Michael and Carolyn. Each time
Carolyn makes this delicious chicken soup, she
is flooded with poignant memories of
when she first met her future husband and his
wonderful mother. I know no other woman
who loved her mother-in-law as much as my
friend loved hers, and making this soup always
honors her mother-in-law's memory.*

Total preparation and
cooking time: 4 hours

Makes 8 servings.

Nutrition information
per serving:

Calories: 356
Fat: 12 g
 Saturated fat: 3.5 g
 Monounsaturated fat: 5 g
Cholesterol: 90 mg
Sodium: 1047 mg
Carbohydrate: 34 g
Fiber: 6 g
Protein: 26 g

2 bouillon cubes, low-sodium
1 medium onion, sliced
1 whole chicken (giblets removed)
6 carrots
3 parsnips
1 medium turnip, sliced
1 bunch Italian parsley (tied together)
1 bunch dill (tied together)
salt/pepper to taste
Manischewitz Matzo Ball and Soup Mix
    Package #2 (or similar soup mix)

Use a large pasta pot with a strainer inside. Fill
it one half to three quarters with water. Bring
the water to a boil, and add the bouillon cubes

and then the onion. The chicken is to be added when the bouillon cubes and the onion reach the boiling point. Skim the residue off the top of the pot after the chicken begins to boil. Add the carrots, parsnips, turnips, parsley, and dill. Lower the flame, leaving the lid half covering the pot. Check it every half hour for 3 hours. After 3 hours, add the soup mix. Stir this into the soup, and boil it an additional hour. Afterward, lift the strainer and separate the chicken bones from the chicken and the vegetables. Fork through the ingredients in the strainer, and remove the bones, skin, parsley, dill, and anything else you don't want to serve in the soup. Add salt and pepper to taste. Put the chicken and vegetables back in the soup, and serve.

Cook's TIP: This chicken soup eats like a meal and tastes great with some crusty bread. It is a bit high in sodium, so you might want to have a smaller portion to minimize your sodium intake.

Main Courses

Tasty Tuna Ties

This quick and easy recipe is a great way to combine complex carbohydrates, lean protein, and vegetables.

Total preparation and
cooking time: 20 minutes

Makes 4 servings.

Nutrition information
per serving:

Calories: 400
Fat: 11 g
  Saturated fat: 1 g
  Monounsaturated fat: 9 g
Cholesterol: 45 mg
Sodium: 540 mg
Carbohydrate: 47 g
Fiber: 2 g
Protein: 29 g

8 ounces bow tie pasta
12.5 ounces canned tuna, chunk white packed in
  water
2 tablespoons red onion, chopped
2 5-inch celery sticks, chopped
¼ cup carrots, shredded
1 teaspoon fresh parsley, chopped
6 tablespoons light mayonnaise

Cook the bow tie pasta, drain, and set aside. In a large bowl, mix the tuna, onion, celery, carrots, parsley, and mayonnaise until all the ingredients are combined. Add the pasta, toss, and serve.

COOK'S TIP: This dish tastes great as a cold pasta salad. You can add corn, chopped tomatoes, or any other vegetables you like.

Fabulous Feta Chicken Salad Sandwich

This is a delicious Greek salad sandwich that incorporates milk, vegetables, and whole grains into your meal. It is very flavorful and filling.

2 ounces grilled chicken, cut into cubes
1½ ounces feta cheese, crumbled
¼ cup red onion, chopped
¼ cup fresh tomatoes, chopped
¼ cup arugula
1 teaspoon balsamic vinegar
3 teaspoons olive oil
pepper to taste (optional)
1 large whole-wheat pita (2 ounces)

Total preparation and cooking time: 15 minutes

Makes 1 serving.

Nutrition information per serving:
Calories: 490
Fat: 25 g
    Saturated fat: 9 g
    Monounsaturated fat: 16 g
Cholesterol: 70 mg
Sodium: 850 mg
Carbohydrate: 43 g
Fiber: 6 g
Protein: 26 g

In a large plastic bag, combine the chicken with the feta cheese, onion, tomatoes, arugula, balsamic vinegar, olive oil, and pepper if desired. Seal the bag and shake it vigorously. Place all the contents into a large bowl. Slice a large, warm pita in half, fill each pocket with chicken mixture, and serve.

COOK'S TIP: This tastes great in a sandwich or as a salad topped with whole-wheat croutons (you can simply toast and chop whole-wheat bread to make them).

Vegetable Mozzarella Pizza

Another great way to pack vegetables into your diet. Although the calories and fat add up since this recipe includes cheese, I prefer the taste of full-fat cheese and will make adjustments during the day to accommodate this and still stay within my daily food plan.

Total preparation and cooking time: 15–20 minutes

Makes 1 serving.

Nutrition information per serving:
Calories: 500
Fat: 27 g
  Saturated fat: 9 g
  Monounsaturated fat: 18 g
Cholesterol: 30 mg
Sodium: 640 mg
Carbohydrate: 46 g
Fiber: 8 g
Protein: 23 g

⅓ cup Japanese eggplant, diced, skin removed
⅓ cup red peppers, diced into ½-inch pieces
⅓ cup tomatoes, diced into ½-inch pieces
1 tablespoon olive oil
½ teaspoon oregano
¼ teaspoon garlic powder
¼ teaspoon cracked pepper
1 large whole-wheat pita, split in half, toasted (2 ounces)
2 ounces part-skim mozzarella cheese, cut in slices

Sauté the eggplant, red peppers, and tomatoes in olive oil with the oregano, garlic powder, and pepper for 8 to 10 minutes. Remove them from the pan and place them in a bowl. Split the whole-wheat pita in half and toast it. Top the pita halves with the vegetable mixture and add sliced mozzarella.

🍴Cook's tip: You can replace any of these vegetables with mushrooms, broccoli, or cauliflower for variety. You can also save some fat by substituting fat-free mozzarella (if you like the taste) or grated parmesan cheese for the part-skim mozzarella.

Molly's Marvelous Lentils

According to my friend Anne Sailer, this recipe was developed out of her need to find foods that were both appealing and easy to eat (and were not a choking hazard) for her then one-year-old daughter, Molly, who at the time refused to eat pureed food. As Anne desperately searched for foods with just the right texture, lentils came to mind. This recipe has grown with Molly, and, according to Anne, it's a "four-season, super-healthy family favorite."

Total preparation and cooking time: 1 hour

Makes 6 servings.

Nutrition information per serving:
Calories: 230
Fat: 3 g
  Saturated fat: 0 g
  Monounsaturated fat: 3 g
Cholesterol: 0 mg
Sodium: 240 mg
Carbohydrate: 41 g
Fiber: 11 g
Protein: 13 g

1 tablespoon extra-virgin olive oil
1 large onion, chopped
1 teaspoon cumin
1 teaspoon cinnamon
½ teaspoon sea salt
1½ cups red lentils
3 cups water
1½ cups carrots, sliced
1½ cups zucchini, sliced
3 cups tomatoes, finely chopped
1 cup currants
1 tablespoon cocoa powder

Heat a large skillet and add the oil. Sauté the onion, cumin, cinnamon, and salt over medium heat until the onion is soft and lightly browned. Add the lentils, water, carrots, zucchini, tomatoes, currants, and cocoa powder, and bring this to a boil. Reduce the heat to low, and simmer for 25 to 30 minutes or until it's the desired consistency.

COOK'S TIP: You can serve this alone as a side dish or over brown or wild rice. You can also wrap the lentils in a warm flour tortilla with melted low-fat cheddar cheese. You may substitute yellow squash, parsnips, and mushrooms for the vegetables and, for special occasions, use French green lentils (they're more expensive and are often used in fine restaurants).

Chicken Quesadilla

This is one of my personal favorites—a great way to fit some lean protein, milk, and vegetables into your diet.

½ pound chicken breasts, skinless and boneless
2 teaspoons light teriyaki sauce, low-sodium
pepper to taste (optional)
1 tablespoon canola oil
nonstick cooking spray
½ cup red peppers, cut in strips
½ cup green peppers, cut in strips
½ cup red onion, sliced
1 tablespoon fresh cilantro, chopped
1 teaspoon chili powder
4 flour tortillas, approximately 1 ounce each
¼ cup shredded low-fat cheddar cheese

Total preparation and cooking time: 30 minutes

Marinating time: 10 minutes

Makes 2 servings.

Nutrition information per serving:
Calories: 450
Fat: 14.5 g
 Saturated fat: 3.0 g
 Monounsaturated fat: 7.0 g
Cholesterol: 69 mg
Sodium: 677 mg
Carbohydrate: 42 g
Fiber: 4 g
Protein: 36 g

Cut the chicken breasts into thin strips. Place in a bowl. Add teriyaki sauce and pepper (if desired) and combine them so that the teriyaki covers all the chicken strips evenly. Heat a large skillet on medium heat with 1 tablespoon of canola oil. At the same time, preheat the oven to 375 degrees F and spray the nonstick cooking spray on a large baking sheet. When

the oil gets hot in the skillet, add the chicken
and sauté for 2 minutes. Then add the red
peppers, green peppers, red onion, cilantro,
and chili powder, and stir for 3 to 4 minutes
until the vegetables are wilted. When the
chicken and vegetables are thoroughly
cooked, place them in a bowl and blot them
with paper towels to remove excess oil. When
the oven is heated, place 2 flour tortillas side
by side on the baking sheet. Add the chicken
and vegetables to each tortilla and sprinkle
with cheddar cheese. Then cover each with a
flour tortilla to make quesadillas. Bake them
for about 8 minutes or until golden brown.

Cook's TIP: These taste great served with
salsa or reduced-fat sour cream. To serve as
an appetizer, cut the quesadillas into triangles.
To save time (and oil), you can grill the
chicken. This recipe can also be made with a
lean meat like flank steak.

Fast Chili

*Chili, onions, and kidney beans are loaded
with nutrients. This dish is quick and easy and
has less fat, sodium, and calories than traditional chili.*

½ pound lean ground beef
¼ cup minced onion
1½ tablespoons chili powder
¼ teaspoon ground cumin
15½ ounces kidney beans, canned and drained
    (save ⅓ cup of the liquid)
1 cup canned tomato puree, no salt added

Total preparation and
cooking time: 20 minutes

Makes 4 servings.

Nutrition information
per serving:
Calories: 210
Fat: 3.5 g
  Saturated fat: 1 g
  Monounsaturated fat: 1 g
Cholesterol: 30 mg
Sodium: 310 mg
Carbohydrate: 32 g
Fiber: 12 g
Protein: 20 g

Cook the beef in a large nonstick skillet until
it's lightly browned. Drain off the fat and set
aside. In the same skillet, cook the onion, chili
powder, and cumin until tender, for 1 to 2
minutes, stirring occasionally. Add the beans,
bean liquid, tomato purée, and beef. Bring this
to a boil over high heat. Reduce the heat to
medium-low and simmer, covered, for 10
minutes.

Cook's TIP: This chili tastes great with a
mixed green salad with light dressing, a
whole-grain roll, and pineapple chunks for
dessert (the vitamin C in the pineapple will
enhance the absorption of iron from the beef).

Nana Burgers

*Memories of my childhood include devouring
many a Nana Burger cooked by none other
than my mother's mother. Even though Nana is
no longer with us, it seems like only yesterday*

when my parents, my older brother, and I drove on weekends from Long Island to Brooklyn, New York, to visit Nana and Papa. We'd walk into their apartment and be overcome by the delicious aromas of Nana's cooking. When we bit into her burgers and other delights, we could just taste the love.

Total preparation and cooking time: 30 minutes

Makes 4 servings.

Nutrition information per serving:
Calories: 270
Fat: 15 g
 Saturated fat: 3.5 g
 Monounsaturated fat: 5 g
Cholesterol: 60 mg
Sodium: 570 mg
Carbohydrate: 11 g
Fiber: 1 g
Protein: 24 g

1 pound of lean ground sirloin
¼ cup red onion, finely chopped
3 cloves garlic, finely chopped
⅓ cup matzo meal
1 egg
3 teaspoons Dijon mustard
½ teaspoon dried oregano
¾ teaspoon salt
pepper to taste
3 tablespoons peanut oil

In a large bowl combine the sirloin, onion, garlic, matzo meal, egg, mustard, oregano, salt, and pepper; mix well. Form the mixture into 4 patties; set them aside. In a large non-stick skillet, heat the peanut oil over medium heat. Add the patties, and cook them 4 to 5 minutes on each side, 4 minutes for medium and 5 minutes for medium-well. Remove the patties, and drain on paper towels.

Cook's tip: When you mold the patties, be sure not to make them too flat or compact because then they will taste dry. Instead, make them plumper (this will help them stay moist and juicy). You can also substitute ground white meat chicken or turkey for the sirloin.

Crunchy Chicken Nuggets

These chicken nuggets are a timeless favorite for parents and kids alike. Both of my boys devour these, though my younger son gets more excited by them—he dips them in grated parmesan cheese during dinner and loves to eat them cold for lunch the next day!

nonstick cooking spray
1 pound chicken breast, skinless and boneless
2 cups corn flakes cereal
½ cup bread crumbs
¼ cup parmesan cheese
½ teaspoon garlic powder
½ teaspoon onion powder
4 egg whites
1 tablespoon olive oil

Total preparation and cooking time: 30 minutes

Makes 4 servings.

Nutrition information per serving:
Calories: 310
Fat: 9 g
 Saturated fat: 2 g
 Monounsaturated fat: 7 g
Cholesterol: 70 mg
Sodium: 410 mg
Carbohydrate: 23 g
Fiber: 1 g
Protein: 35 g

Preheat the oven to 350 degrees F. Use nonstick cooking spray to coat a nonstick baking sheet, and set it aside. Divide the chicken breast into 8 even pieces. Pour the corn flakes, breadcrumbs, parmesan cheese, garlic powder, and onion powder into a large plastic bag. Seal the bag, removing most of the air, and mash the ingredients until fine. Pour the mixture onto a large plate. Beat the egg whites and olive oil in a medium bowl. Dip the chicken into the egg-and-olive-oil mixture and then into the cornflake mixture, coating each piece completely. Place the coated chicken pieces onto a baking sheet. Bake for 8 to 10 minutes. Serve.

COOK'S TIP: This chicken goes well with roasted red potatoes and a green vegetable. It can also be sliced and served cold to top salad greens. To make this into a flavorful appetizer,

cut the chicken into bite-sized pieces and add
½ cup of finely chopped raw cashews to the
corn flake and bread crumb mixture.

Olive and Sun-Dried Tomato Pasta

*This recipe, created by my dad, is flavorful and
hearty. Because my dad delights in sharing his
great love of food with family and friends, you
can imagine how pleased he was when my son
Eli not only tried this dish, but ate it at the age
of two!*

4 cups whole-wheat penne
12 sun-dried tomatoes (packed in oil), diced
4 cloves fresh garlic, finely chopped
12 large black pitted olives, sliced
4 tablespoons fresh parsley
1 teaspoon dried oregano
8 teaspoons olive oil
¼ cup dry Spanish sherry
½ cup pasta water

Total preparation and cooking time: 30 minutes

Makes 4 servings.

Nutrition information per serving:
Calories: 330
Fat: 11 g
  Saturated fat: 1.5 g
  Monounsaturated fat: 9.5 g
Cholesterol: 0 mg
Sodium: 250 mg
Carbohydrate: 48 g
Fiber: 3 g
Protein: 9 g

Cook the penne according to the package
directions and set it aside (save ½ cup of the
leftover pasta water). Blot the sun-dried tomatoes with paper towels to remove excess oil. In
a large bowl, combine the sun-dried tomatoes,
garlic, black olives, parsley, oregano, olive oil,
sherry, and the pasta water. Mix in the penne,
and serve it in small bowls.

COOK'S TIP: You can add diced grilled
chicken to this dish to make it a more complete meal.

Chicken and Broccoli Pasta

This pasta dish is light and easy to prepare. It's appealing to people who don't like saucy pasta but still want some flavor. The grated cheese adds a lot of kick to this basic dish.

1¼ pounds skinless, boneless chicken breast
½ teaspoon dried crushed rosemary
½ teaspoon salt
¼ teaspoon pepper
3 tablespoons olive oil
½ cup fresh onion, chopped
2 cloves fresh garlic, chopped
4 cups broccoli florets
8 ounces penne pasta, cooked and drained
½ cup grated parmesan cheese

Total preparation and cooking time: 20 minutes

Makes 4 servings.

Nutrition information per serving:
Calories: 530
Fat: 16 g
  Saturated fat: 4 g
  Monounsaturated fat: 9 g
Cholesterol: 105 mg
Sodium: 560 mg
Carbohydrate: 49 g
Fiber: 4 g
Protein: 47 g

Preheat the grill for direct heat grilling. Sprinkle the tops of the chicken breasts with rosemary, salt, and pepper. Grill 10 to 12 minutes, or until a meat thermometer reads 180 degrees F, turning once. Slice the chicken and set aside. Meanwhile, in a large nonstick skillet, heat 2 tablespoons olive oil over medium-high heat. Cook the onion and garlic until just softened, 1 to 2 minutes. Add the broccoli, tossing to coat. Cook 2 minutes. Reduce the heat to medium-low and cook, covered, for 10 minutes or until the broccoli is tender. Remove the broccoli mixture from the skillet and place in a bowl lined with paper towels to absorb excess oil; remove the paper towels and discard. Add the sliced chicken, pasta, and parmesan cheese. Drizzle with the remaining 1 tablespoon oil, toss, and serve.

COOK'S TIP: This dish can be served as a hot pasta dish or a cold pasta salad. The broccoli florets can easily be replaced by cauliflower, eggplant, or any other vegetable you prefer.

Linda's Chicken Meatballs and Spaghetti

Linda has been my children's babysitter since my older son, Spencer, was born. Her amazingly simple recipe is delicious. My younger son, Eli, devours this dish and loves to smother his meatballs with extra grated parmesan cheese.

16 ounces lean ground chicken
¼ cup breadcrumbs, seasoned
¼ cup red onion, finely chopped
1 clove garlic, minced
2 tablespoons fresh parsley
¼ teaspoon kosher salt
¼ teaspoon pepper
2 cups tomato sauce (from a jar)
8 ounces (½ box) thin spaghetti, cooked
¼ cup grated parmesan cheese

Total preparation and cooking time: 45 minutes

Makes 4 servings.

Nutrition information per serving:
Calories: 450
Fat: 12 g
  Saturated fat: 2.5 g
  Monounsaturated fat: .5 g
Cholesterol: 80 mg
Sodium: 1,060 mg
Carbohydrate: 58 g
Fiber: 4 g
Protein: 30 g

In a large bowl, combine the chicken with the breadcrumbs, red onion, garlic, parsley, salt, and pepper until the ingredients are evenly distributed. Form the mixture into 12 meatballs. Set a large pan on medium to high heat. Add the tomato sauce and bring it to a boil. When the sauce is boiling, put the meatballs in, lower the flame, and cover. Cook for 10 to 15 minutes. Add the sauce and meatballs to the spaghetti, top it with 1 tablespoon of grated cheese, and serve with the extra grated cheese on the side.

COOK'S TIP: This recipe is admittedly high in sodium, but you can lower its sodium content substantially (without altering the flavor too much) if you use low-sodium tomato sauce and/or skip the salt. The meatballs can also be sliced and served cold on whole-grain bread for lunch the next day.

Penne with Olives and Sausage

This is one of my dad's favorite dishes to make. The combination of chicken sausage, sun-dried tomatoes, and olives adds a unique texture and gives this dish a punchy flavor.

1 pound (1 box) penne pasta
1 cup pasta water
1 pound Italian-style chicken sausage
10 cloves of garlic, diced
¼ cup sun-dried tomatoes in oil, drained, julienned
¼ cup extra-virgin olive oil
1 15-ounce can black pitted olives
1 teaspoon dried oregano
2 tablespoons parsley, chopped
¼ teaspoon red pepper flakes
salt and pepper to taste

Total preparation and cooking time: 25 minutes

Makes 8 servings.

Nutrition information per serving:
Calories: 413
Fat: 19 g
  Saturated fat: 3 g
  Monounsaturated fat: 9.5 g
Cholesterol: 37 mg
Sodium: 727 mg
Carbohydrate: 51 g
Fiber: 5 g
Protein: 15 g

Cook the penne according to the package directions and set it aside (save 1 cup of the pasta water). Grill the sausages for 8 minutes, and slice them into pieces. Sauté the garlic and sun-dried tomatoes in olive oil. Do not burn the garlic. Add the olives, oregano, parsley, and red pepper flakes, and simmer for 5 minutes. Add the cooked penne, the pasta water, salt, and pepper. Stir and serve immediately.

COOK'S TIP: Instead of salt and pepper, you can add Cajun seasoning to give this dish a great ethnic flavor.

Lemon Garlic Chicken

This marinade that my mom makes for her chicken takes the cake. It is truly the best I've had.

1 pound chicken breasts, skinless and boneless, cut into 4 pieces
lemon juice (from 1½ fresh lemons)
1 lemon rind, grated
3 cloves fresh garlic
1 tablespoon fresh parsley, chopped
1 tablespoon ground cilantro
2 tablespoons olive oil
nonstick cooking spray

Cut the chicken into 4 pieces. Blend the lemon juice, lemon rind, garlic, parsley, cilantro, and olive oil in a large bowl. Put the chicken breasts into the bowl and coat them with the marinade. Cover the chicken, and refrigerate it for 1 hour. Grill for 5 minutes or so on each side, or coat a nonstick skillet with cooking spray and sauté the chicken on medium heat for 3 to 4 minutes on each side or until thoroughly cooked. Serve.

Cook's tip: This chicken can be served hot with broccoli, brussels sprouts, or green beans or cold and sliced over salad greens.

Total preparation and cooking time: 1 hour, 20 minutes

Marinating time: 1 hour.

Makes 4 servings.

Nutrition information per serving:
Calories: 190
Fat: 8 g
  Saturated fat: 1.5 g
  Monounsaturated fat: 7.5 g
Cholesterol: 65 mg
Sodium: 75 mg
Carbohydrate: 2 g
Fiber: 0 g
Protein: 26 g

Baked Cod Fish

This is a great way to get those heart-healthy omega-3 fats into your diet. The breadcrumbs add a crunchy texture to the fish and make this a great dish for kids, packed with protein and other key nutrients.

1 pound cod fish
1 cup corn flakes
¼ cup seasoned bread crumbs
½ teaspoon garlic powder
1 teaspoon paprika
½ teaspoon onion powder
1 tablespoon fresh parsley
½ teaspoon kosher salt
¼ teaspoon pepper
2 large egg whites, raw
nonstick cooking spray
lemon wedges

Total preparation and cooking time: 30 minutes

Makes 4 servings.

Nutrition information per serving:
Calories: 190
Fat: 1.5 g
  Saturated fat: 0 g
  Monounsaturated fat: 0 g
Cholesterol: 60 mg
Sodium: 600 mg
Carbohydrate: 12 g
Fiber: 1 g
Protein: 31 g

Preheat the oven to 400 degrees F. Divide the fish into 4 even pieces. Pour the corn flakes cereal, bread crumbs, garlic powder, paprika, onion powder, parsley, salt, and pepper into a large plastic bag. Seal the bag, removing most of the air, and mash the cereal with your fist until the cereal is fine. Pour the cereal and bread crumb mixture onto a large plate. Crack the eggs into a bowl, removing the yolks, and set aside. First dip each piece of cod in enough egg to evenly coat it, and then dip it into the cereal and breadcrumb mixture. Repeat for each piece of fish. Use nonstick cooking spray to coat a nonstick baking sheet, and place the fish on the baking sheet. Bake for 8 to 10 minutes. Serve with lemon wedges.

COOK'S TIP: For the breadcrumbs, you can use any seasoned brand. However, Japanese breadcrumbs—panko breadcrumbs—are made from rice and impart great flavor and texture to this baked fish dish. This cereal and breadcrumb mixture can also be used to coat chicken or eggplant.

Sensational Salmon

This recipe, created by my friend Halee, is easy to prepare, and the combination of ingredients makes the salmon (rich in heart-healthy omega-3 fats), moist and flavorful.

3 mushrooms, chopped
4 black olives, chopped
⅛ cup fresh tomatoes, chopped
4 ounces salmon
nonstick olive oil–flavored cooking spray
1 tablespoon honey mustard
1 bay leaf
¼ teaspoon salt
pepper (to taste)
rosemary (to taste)
2 tablespoons white wine

Total preparation and cooking time: 20 to 30 minutes

Makes 1 serving.

Nutrition information per serving:
Calories: 290
Fat: 15 g
  Saturated fat: 3 g
  Monounsaturated fat: 12 g
Cholesterol: 65 mg
Sodium: 930 mg
Carbohydrate: 10 g
Fiber: 1 g
Protein: 24 g

Preheat the oven to 350 degrees F. In a small bowl, combine the mushrooms, black olives, and tomatoes, and add the mixture to the salmon. Set it aside. Cover a baking sheet with aluminum foil. Spray another piece of foil with the cooking spray, and put it on top of the baking sheet. Place the salmon in the middle of the sheet of foil. Spread the honey mustard on top of the salmon. Raise the sides of the foil around the salmon. Add the vegetable mixture to the salmon, along with the bay leaf, salt, pepper, and rosemary. Pour the white wine on the salmon. Fold and seal tight the packet surrounding the fish. Bake it for 20 to 25 minutes. Remove the bay leaf before serving.

COOK's TIP: Instead of white wine, you can use balsamic vinegar to give the salmon a tangy taste. You could also replace the mushrooms with shredded cabbage, carrots, or red bell peppers.

Asian Crab Cakes

According to my dad, a wonderful cook, Vietnamese chili garlic sauce lends great flavor and an Asian flare to this traditional seafood dish.

1 slice whole-wheat bread
1 pound lump crab meat
½ cup light mayonnaise
2 eggs
2 tablespoons Dijon mustard
2 tablespoons lemon juice
¼ teaspoon salt
1 tablespoon sesame oil
1 tablespoon Vietnamese chili garlic sauce
¼ cup peanut oil

Total preparation and cooking time: 1 hour, 10 minutes

Makes 6 servings.

Nutrition information per serving:
Calories: 240
Fat: 17 g
  Saturated fat: 2.5 g
  Monounsaturated fat: 7 g
Cholesterol: 125 mg
Sodium: 605 mg
Carbohydrate: 4 g
Fiber: 0 g
Protein: 19 g

Toast 1 slice of whole-wheat bread and pulverize it in a food processor for 1 minute. Set this aside in a cup. Lightly fold together the crab meat, mayonnaise, eggs, ½ cup of breadcrumbs, Dijon mustard, lemon juice, salt, sesame oil, and chili garlic sauce. Refrigerate this for 1 hour. Form the mixture by hand into 6 small cakes. Dip each one into the remaining ¼ cup of breadcrumbs. Sauté the crab cakes in peanut oil for 1 minute on each side over medium heat.

COOK'S TIP: You can make these crab cakes into bite-sized pieces and serve them as an appetizer. They also taste great served warm over salad greens with a light vinaigrette dressing.

Broiled Sesame Fish

Pairing fish with sesame seeds and parsley creates a great texture and flavor.

1 pound cod fillets, fresh or frozen
1 teaspoon trans fat–free margarine, melted
1 tablespoon lemon juice
1 teaspoon dried tarragon leaves
⅛ teaspoon salt
dash of pepper
1 tablespoon sesame seeds
1 tablespoon parsley, chopped

Total preparation and cooking time: 30 minutes

Makes 4 servings.

Nutrition information per serving:
Calories: 110
Fat: 2.5 g
  Saturated fat: 0 g
  Monounsaturated fat: 0.5 g
Cholesterol: 45 mg
Sodium: 150 mg
Carbohydrate: 1 g
Fiber: 0 g
Protein: 19 g

Thaw the frozen cod fish in the refrigerator overnight or defrost it briefly in a microwave oven. Cut the fish into 4 portions. Place the fish on a broiler pan lined with aluminum foil. Brush the margarine over the fish. Mix together the lemon juice, tarragon, salt, and pepper. Pour this over the fish. Sprinkle the sesame seeds evenly over the fish. Broil it for 12 minutes, or until the fish flakes easily with a fork—about 12 minutes. Garnish it with parsley.

Cook's tip: This fish goes well with wild rice and a green vegetable.

Tofu Teriyaki Stir-Fry

This flavorful, hearty dish is a great way to incorporate vegetables and protein into your diet. It also helps you meet your weekly quota for beans to boost your nutrient intake.

8 ounces firm tofu, cut into cubes
2 tablespoons light teriyaki sauce
3 tablespoons olive oil
2 garlic cloves, chopped
1 cup carrots, chopped
2 cups green beans, chopped
2 cups broccoli florets, chopped
½ cup bamboo shoots
½ cup water
4 scallions, sliced
2 teaspoons roasted sesame oil
1 teaspoon onion powder

Total preparation and cooking time: 40 minutes

Marinating time: 10 minutes

Makes 4 servings.

Nutrition information per serving:
Calories: 220
Fat: 16 g
　Saturated fat: 2 g
　Monounsaturated fat: 14 g
Cholesterol: 0 mg
Sodium: 260 mg
Carbohydrate: 15 g
Fiber: 5 g
Protein: 9 g

Marinate the tofu with 1 tablespoon of light teriyaki sauce for 10 minutes. Add 1 tablespoon of olive oil to the skillet, and heat on medium heat. Add the tofu and brown it for 5 to 6 minutes. Remove the tofu and set it aside. Add 2 tablespoons of olive oil and the garlic and carrots to a wok or a pan and stir-fry for 1 minute. Then add the beans, broccoli, bamboo shoots, 1 tablespoon of the teriyaki sauce, and ½ cup of water. Cover it, lower the heat, and cook for 4 minutes. Remove the lid and add the scallions. When it's cooked, place the mixture in a large bowl. Add the tofu, roasted sesame oil, and onion powder. Toss and serve.

COOK'S TIP: The roasted sesame oil, drizzled on just before serving, adds a lot of flavor and richness to this vegetarian dish.

Super Steak

This recipe is packed with iron, but the addition of tomatoes makes it a good source of vitamins A and C and lycopene. It also has a nice blend of seasonings and spices that adds some spunk to steak.

¾ pound beef round steak, boneless
½ cup celery, sliced
1 tablespoon onion, chopped
1 tablespoon flour
1 16-ounce can of tomatoes, no salt added
2 tablespoons water
1 tablespoon parsley, chopped
1 tablespoon soy sauce, low-sodium
½ teaspoon ginger root, minced
¼ teaspoon salt
⅛ teaspoon garlic, ground
⅛ teaspoon red pepper flakes
1 bay leaf, chopped

Total preparation and cooking time: 1 hour

Makes 4 servings.

Nutrition information per serving:
Calories: 220
Fat: 8 g
  Saturated fat: 2.5 g
  Monounsaturated fat: 3 g
Cholesterol: 85 mg
Sodium: 220 mg
Carbohydrate: 7 g
Fiber: 1 g
Protein: 30 g

Trim all of the fat from the steak. Slice it across the grain diagonally into thin strips. Heat a nonstick frying pan; cook the steak, celery, and onion until the steak is browned. Drain off the fat. Stir the flour into the beef mixture. Add the tomatoes, water, parsley, soy sauce, ginger root, salt, garlic, red pepper flakes, and bay leaf. Bring this to a boil; reduce the heat, cover, and cook over low heat for 40 minutes or until the meat is tender. Remove the bay leaf and serve.

COOK'S TIP: This dish works well over rice or noodles.

Vegetable Turkey Chili

This recipe, from Linda, one of our oldest family friends, is simple to prepare and helps you pack lots of vegetables into a single meal.

½ cup onions, chopped
2 tablespoons olive oil
3 cloves garlic, minced
1 pound ground turkey
1 8-ounce can whole tomatoes or fresh, chopped
1 tablespoon chili powder
½ cup carrots, chopped
½ cup celery, chopped
½ cup red pepper, sliced
1 cup green beans, chopped

Total preparation and cooking time: 1 hour, 15 minutes

Makes 4 servings.

Nutrition information per serving:
Calories: 340
Fat: 24 g
    Saturated fat: 6 g
    Monounsaturated fat: 6 g
Cholesterol: 75 mg
Sodium: 240 mg
Carbohydrate: 12 g
Fiber: 4 g
Protein: 20 g

In a nonstick pan, brown the onions in the olive oil for 4 minutes on medium heat. Add the garlic and cook for 1 minute. Add the turkey, and brown it for 4 minutes. Add the tomatoes, chili powder, carrots, celery, and red peppers. Cover and let it simmer on a low heat for 45 minutes. Add the green beans, cover, and cook for 10 minutes.

COOK'S TIP: You can substitute ground veal, chicken, or beef for the ground turkey. This chili can be eaten as a main dish, or it can top pasta.

Sauces

Vegetable and Bean Tomato Sauce

This flavorful recipe, courtesy of my friend Keri, combines all the best that the plant world has to offer—an abundance of flavorful, nutrient-packed vegetables and beans. It has a great texture and can be used to complement pasta or even chicken dishes.

1 tablespoon olive oil
2 medium ripe tomatoes
4 shitake mushrooms, thinly sliced
2 ounces portobello mushrooms, thinly sliced
½ small zucchini, thinly sliced
1 cup canned black beans, low-sodium, drained and rinsed
1 teaspoon fresh basil, chopped
½ Italian eggplant, chopped

Total preparation and cooking time: 30 minutes

Makes 2 servings.

Nutrition information per serving:
Calories: 110
Fat: 4 g
　Saturated fat: 0 g
　Monounsaturated fat: 4 g
Cholesterol: 0 mg
Sodium: 135 mg
Carbohydrate: 19 g
Fiber: 6 g
Protein: 4 g

Add the olive oil to a saucepan and heat it on medium. Chop the tomatoes into medium-sized pieces. Put them into the saucepan. Add the mushrooms, zucchini, black beans, and basil. Simmer, and stir constantly so that it doesn't stick. Add the eggplant. Once the mixture starts to lightly boil, lower the flame and cover. Cook it for about 20 minutes, or until the tomatoes and vegetables are soft but not overcooked. If the ingredients stick together or if they're not saucy enough, add some vegetable broth or water.

COOK'S TIP: This sauce tastes great over whole-wheat pasta and with a few sprinkles of parmesan cheese. You can substitute asparagus or broccoli for some or all of the vegetables, though these should be steamed, then added to the sauce once it's completely cooked. Baby spinach can also be added to the sauce 2 minutes prior to completion.

Terrific Tomato Sauce

I know firsthand that my dad's tomato sauce is indeed sensational. He says that because this tomato sauce is so quick and easy to make, yet tastes so good, it's "a pleasant surprise to anyone who thinks good tomato sauce can only be made by a grandma who slaves over the stove for eight hours."

4 garlic cloves, finely diced
2 tablespoons extra-virgin olive oil
¼ cup sun-dried tomatoes, in oil, drained and cut into strips
¼ teaspoon red pepper flakes (optional)
1 28-ounce can diced imported Italian tomatoes, no sugar added
¼ cup fresh parsley, chopped
salt to taste (optional)

Total preparation and cooking time: 15 minutes

Makes 4 servings.

Nutrition information per serving:
Calories: 160
Fat: 8 g
   Saturated fat: 1 g
   Monounsaturated fat: 6 g
Cholesterol: 0 mg
Sodium: 790 mg (does not include added salt)
Carbohydrate: 19 g
Fiber: 2 g
Protein: 2 g

Sauté the garlic, oil, sun-dried tomatoes, and pepper on high heat for 2 minutes. Add the tomatoes, and cook over high heat for 5 more minutes, stirring often. Turn the heat to low, cover the pan, and let it simmer for 5 minutes. Add the parsley and salt to taste. Stir it just before removing it from the heat. Use the sauce immediately, or refrigerate it for later use.

COOK'S TIP: This sauce tastes great over pasta sprinkled with basil and some fresh grated parmesan cheese, with meatballs, or on top of grilled chicken.

Turkey Bolognese Sauce

This tasty sauce, made by my friend Halee, has a great texture and is a great way to add vegetables loaded with vitamin C and fiber to a meal.

olive oil spray
½ teaspoon garlic, chopped
¼ sweet or Vidalia onion, finely chopped
½ large zucchini, chopped
1 medium red pepper, chopped
½ pound ground turkey
2 cups chopped tomatoes
¼ cup white cooking wine
10 large black olives (without pits)
4 small asparagus spears, chopped
2 bay leaves
salt and pepper to taste (optional)

Total preparation and cooking time: 40-45 minutes

Makes 4 servings.

Nutrition information per serving:
Calories: 170
Fat: 11 g
  Saturated fat: 3 g
  Monounsaturated fat: 4 g
Cholesterol: 40 mg
Sodium: 250 mg
Carbohydrate: 9 g
Fiber: 2 g
Protein: 11 g

Heat a large skillet and spray on a coating of olive oil spray; add ½ teaspoon of chopped garlic. When the pan is hot, add the onions, zucchini, and red pepper. Sauté for 5 minutes until they're golden brown. Add the turkey, and sauté another 5 minutes or until everything is thoroughly cooked. Add the tomato, wine, olives, asparagus, and bay leaves. Cover, and set it on low heat. Simmer for 20 minutes. Add salt and pepper to taste.

Cook's tip: You can experiment with different herbs (for example, basil or rosemary). This sauce tastes great over whole-wheat pasta or spaghetti squash.

Side Dishes

Roasted Red Potatoes

The scallions in this recipe add a splash of color, texture, and pizzazz to one of my family's favorite side dishes.

2 pounds red baby creamer potatoes
¼ cup olive oil
2 tablespoons balsamic vinegar
2 cloves fresh garlic, sliced
4 scallions, chopped
½ teaspoon sea salt
¼ teaspoon cracked pepper
1 teaspoon fresh rosemary

Preheat the oven to 400 degrees F. Cut each potato in half. Put the potatoes in a large plastic bag. Add the olive oil, 1 tablespoon of vinegar, garlic, 3 tablespoons of scallions, sea salt, pepper, and rosemary, and seal the bag (try to remove as much air as possible). Shake the bag vigorously so that the ingredients distribute evenly onto the potatoes. Pour the potatoes and mixture onto a nonstick baking pan. Bake for 1 hour, and toss every 20 minutes. Remove from the oven when a fork can easily pierce the potatoes. The potatoes will be dark and crunchy on the outside, yet tender on the inside. Remove the garlic slices, if desired. Before serving, splash the remaining balsamic vinegar on the potatoes, and garnish with 1 tablespoon of scallions.

Cook's tip: If you want a milder taste, you can skip the balsamic vinegar in this recipe or forgo the sea salt if you're watching your

---

Total preparation and cooking time: 1 hour, 15 minutes

Makes 6 servings.

Nutrition information per serving:
Calories: 200
Fat: 9 g
    Saturated fat: 1.5 g
    Monounsaturated fat: 7.5 g
Cholesterol: 0 mg
Sodium: 280 mg
Carbohydrate: 26 g
Fiber: 3 g
Protein: 3 g

sodium intake. This dish is a great accompaniment to chicken, steak, or fish dishes, served with a green vegetable.

Apple Coleslaw

My mom's delicious coleslaw has a lot of crunch, and the addition of apple cider vinegar and sugar gives it a sweet yet tangy flavor.

1½ cups cabbage, shredded
½ cup carrots, shredded
2 tablespoons 1% buttermilk
1 tablespoon apple cider vinegar
½ teaspoon sugar
¼ teaspoon salt
1 tablespoon light mayonnaise

Total preparation and cooking time: 5 minutes

Makes 2 servings.

Nutrition information per serving:
Calories: 60
Fat: 3 g
  Saturated fat: 0 g
  Monounsaturated fat: 1 g
Cholesterol: 5 mg
Sodium: 400 mg
Carbohydrate: 8 g
Fiber: 2 g
Protein: 1 g

Place the cabbage, carrots, buttermilk, apple cider vinegar, sugar, and salt in a large bowl. Add the mayonnaise, and combine all the ingredients. Chill and serve.

Cook's tip: This tastes great as a tuna, turkey, or chicken breast sandwich filler or on its own as a side dish. It can also add crunch to a traditional garden salad.

Garlic Brussels Sprouts

I love these as prepared by my dad, but minus the pepper. They have a great texture and bring a lot of flavor to any meal.

2 cups raw brussels sprouts
2 tablespoons olive oil
2 cloves of garlic
4 sun-dried tomatoes (packed in oil)
⅛ teaspoon of salt
pepper to taste

Add 2 cups of water to a pot, and bring it to a boil. Cut the root ends off the brussels sprouts, then cut the sprouts into halves. Add the brussels sprouts to the water, and boil for 4 to 5 minutes. Remove, and place them in a bowl of ice-cold water to stop their cooking. Remove from the water and blot with paper towels. Heat the olive oil in a skillet. Add the garlic and sauté for 1 minute. Add the brussels sprouts, and sauté for 2 to 3 minutes until cooked. Remove them from the heat, and place them in a bowl. Toss in the sun-dried tomatoes, and add salt and pepper to taste. Serve.

Cook's tip: You can have these as a side dish for beef, chicken, or broiled fish. They can also be served with a vegetable burger or be used to top a pasta like penne or ziti.

Total preparation and cooking time: 25 to 30 minutes

Makes 2 servings.

Nutrition information per serving:
Calories: 170
Fat: 14 g
  Saturated fat: 2 g
  Monounsaturated fat: 12 g
Cholesterol: 0 mg
Sodium: 250 mg
Carbohydrate: 11 g
Fiber: 4 g
Protein: 4 g

Asparagus and Mushrooms with Fresh Coriander

This is the favorite recipe of one of our old family friends, Linda. The fresh coriander and other ingredients give this simple dish a lot of flavor and make it a terrific-tasting side dish that melts in your mouth.

1 pound fresh thin asparagus
1 cup chicken bouillon or broth, low-sodium
½ pound fresh mushrooms, sliced
2 tablespoon shallots, sliced
4 tablespoon fresh coriander leaves, chopped
pepper to taste

Total preparation and cooking time: 20 minutes

Makes 4 servings.

Nutrition information per serving:
Calories: 50
Fat: 0.5 g
  Saturated fat: 0 g
  Monounsaturated fat: 0 g
Cholesterol: 0 mg
Sodium: 25 mg
Carbohydrate: 8 g
Fiber: 3 g
Protein: 6 g

Cut the asparagus in 1-inch pieces, and set them aside. Heat the bouillon in a skillet. Add the mushrooms, and sauté on high heat for 4 minutes. Add the asparagus and shallots, and cook for 4 minutes. Add the coriander and pepper. Toss the ingredients together and serve.

Cook's tip: This tastes great as a side dish with chicken or lean beef, but it can also work well over pasta with some grated parmesan cheese.

Halee's Mashed Butternut Squash

The addition of maple syrup at the end gives this recipe a sweet kick. My friend Halee, who created this recipe, loves to eat this dish alongside chicken and notes that it's an easy way to add a vegetable at dinner.

1 butternut squash
2 tablespoons trans fat–free margarine
1 teaspoon cinnamon
1 teaspoon maple syrup

Total preparation and cooking time: 45 minutes to 1 hour

Makes 4 servings.

Nutrition information per serving:
Calories: 110
Fat: 6 g
  Saturated fat: 1 g
  Monounsaturated fat: 2.5 g
Cholesterol: 0 mg
Sodium: 80 mg
Carbohydrate: 16 g
Fiber: 4 g
Protein: 2 g

Preheat the oven to 400 degrees F. Split the squash in half. Scoop out the seeds. Place the squash, skin side down, on an aluminum foil–covered cookie sheet. Spread 1 tablespoon of the margarine on each half of the squash. Sprinkle ½ teaspoon of cinnamon on each half of the squash. Wrap the squash in the foil, and place it in the oven. Bake it for 45 minutes or until soft. Remove it from the oven, and let it cool for 5 minutes. Scoop out the inside of the squash, and place this in a bowl. Mash it in the maple syrup, and serve.

COOK'S TIP: If you have high cholesterol, you can easily use Benecol, a cholesterol-lowering butter substitute, instead of the trans fat–free margarine in this recipe without substantially altering the great flavor of the dish.

Alpine Swiss Chard with Raisins and Pine Nuts

My dad loves this side dish so much that he sometimes has it as a main course. The Swiss chard gives this recipe a robust flavor, and it's loaded with vitamins A and C, as well as fiber.

1 pound Swiss chard, cleaned
3 cloves garlic, diced
2 tablespoons extra-virgin olive oil
1 ounce pine nuts
½ cup raisins
¼ teaspoon salt (optional)
pepper, a dash (optional)

Cut the Swiss chard into thin strips and remove the veins. Sauté the garlic in olive oil over medium heat. Add the Swiss chard and cook for 3 minutes or until tender. Add the pine nuts, raisins, salt, and pepper, and heat for 2 minutes until thoroughly cooked.

Cook's tip: This makes a great side dish for chicken or fish.

Total preparation and cooking time: 15 minutes

Makes 4 servings.

Nutrition information per serving (includes ¼ teaspoon salt):
Calories: 240
Fat: 16 g
   Saturated fat: 3 g
   Monounsaturated fat: 8 g
Cholesterol: 0 mg
Sodium: 250 mg
Carbohydrate: 21 g
Fiber: 4 g
Protein: 5 g

Sweet Potato French Fries

This delicious recipe is courtesy of my friend Dave. It is easy to make and is a great way to serve up a deep-orange vegetable that's loaded with vitamin A and rich in fiber.

2 medium sweet potatoes, cleaned and unpeeled
4 sprays nonstick canola oil spray
1 tablespoon olive oil
¼ teaspoon salt
½ teaspoon black pepper
½ teaspoon onion powder
½ teaspoon garlic powder
cayenne pepper (optional)

Total preparation and cooking time: 50 minutes

Makes 2 servings.

Nutrition information per serving:
Calories: 200
Fat: 10 g
  Saturated fat: 1 g
  Monounsaturated fat: 6 g
Cholesterol: 0 mg
Sodium: 330 mg
Carbohydrate: 28 g
Fiber: 4 g
Protein: 2 g

Slice the unpeeled potatoes into thick matchsticks. Spray a cookie sheet with the nonstick spray. Arrange the potatoes on the cookie sheet and lightly brush on the olive oil. Sprinkle the potatoes with salt, pepper, onion powder, and garlic powder. For an added zing, sprinkle on a dash of cayenne pepper. Bake the potatoes in the oven at 400 degrees F for approximately 40 minutes or until tender (they are easily pierced with a fork). Set the oven to broil, and brown them until their tops are golden brown.

COOK'S TIP: These taste great with virtually any fish, chicken, or lean meat dish.

Sweets and Treats

Mango-Banana Smoothie

The honey gives this smoothie a kick, and the frozen fruit makes it creamy like a milkshake.

½ cup fresh frozen banana
½ cup nonfat yogurt
½ cup fresh mango, cubed
1 teaspoon vanilla extract
1 teaspoon honey

Wrap a ripe banana in plastic wrap and freeze it overnight. Blend the yogurt, mango, frozen banana, vanilla extract, and honey in a blender until smooth. Chill or serve immediately.

Cook's tip: You can replace the mango or frozen banana with any ripe fruit, such as peaches, nectarines, strawberries, or blueberries.

Total preparation and cooking time: 5 minutes

Makes 1 serving.

Nutrition information per serving:
Calories: 200
Fat: 0 g
 Saturated fat: 0 g
 Monounsaturated fat: 0 g
Cholesterol: 5 mg
Sodium: 70 mg
Carbohydrate: 47 g
Fiber: 3 g
Protein: 6 g

Oatmeal Applesauce Cookies

Applesauce lends a moist texture to these cookies. And what a great way to get some oatmeal—a whole grain—into your day!

nonstick cooking spray
1½ cups rolled oats
1 cup unbleached all-purpose flour
½ teaspoon ground allspice
¼ teaspoon baking soda
¼ teaspoon salt
6 tablespoons trans fat–free margarine
⅓ cup sugar
⅓ cup light brown sugar
1 egg white
½ cup unsweetened applesauce
½ cup seedless raisins, chopped

Total preparation and cooking time: 30 minutes

Makes 36 cookies.

Nutrition information per serving:
Calories: 60
Fat: 2 g
  Saturated fat: 0 g
  Monounsaturated fat: 1g
Cholesterol: 0 mg
Sodium: 45 mg
Carbohydrate: 10 g
Fiber: 1 g
Protein: 1 g

Preheat the oven to 375 degrees F. Spray a large baking sheet with nonstick cooking spray. In a large bowl, combine the oats, flour, allspice, baking soda, and salt, and set this aside. In another bowl, beat the margarine, sugar, and brown sugar until creamy. Reduce the speed to low and add the egg white, mixing until combined. Alternately, add the flour mixture and the applesauce until just combined. Fold in the raisins. Drop by level tablespoonfuls onto the prepared baking sheet. Bake for 15–17 minutes until the edges are lightly browned. Cool and serve.

Cook's tip: These taste great dunked in skim milk or crumbled onto frozen vanilla yogurt.

Wholesome Sugar Cookies

My friend and Web site designer Anne Sailer told me this story: "One spring, my son Jacob saw Easter cookies in the grocery store and desperately wanted to buy a batch. Knowing those cookies were loaded with white sugar, white flour, and partially hydrogenated oil, I suggested that we race home and bake our own. He was thrilled! I grabbed an old cookbook from the shelf and found a simple sugar cookie recipe, then I altered it to produce a more healthful version for our family. Jacob helped me measure every ingredient and waited with bated breath for the dough to chill. Once the dough was ready, he floured and rolled, and floured and rolled, and used every cookie cutter in the house. The second the cookies came out of the oven, he chose a special one to eat, barely waiting for it to cool. Jacob's wonderful cookies have become a holiday staple in our house, and they're perfect—and low guilt!—for those special afternoons when it's just time to bake cookies."

Total preparation and cooking time: 1½ hours (includes chilling the dough)

Makes 40 servings.

Nutrition information per serving:
Calories: 60
Fat: 3 g
    Saturated fat: 0 g
    Monounsaturated fat: 1 g
Cholesterol: 10 mg
Sodium: 65 mg
Carbohydrate: 7 g
Fiber: 0 g
Protein: 1 g

½ cup trans fat–free margarine
1 tablespoon canola or safflower oil (preferably cold-pressed)
2 eggs (preferably free-range)
⅔ cup natural sugar (turbinado, raw cane, or date)
1 teaspoon vanilla
2 cups whole-wheat pastry flour
1¼ teaspoons baking powder (preferably aluminum-free)
¼ teaspoon sea salt

Cream the margarine, oil, eggs, natural sugar, and vanilla until smooth and light. In a separate bowl, combine the flour, baking powder, and salt, mixing thoroughly to evenly distribute the dry ingredients. Add the dry ingredients to the wet ingredients, and mix thoroughly. Chill the dough for at least a half-hour. Roll the dough on a well-floured board to ¼-inch thick; cut it with cookie cutters and place the shapes on a cookie sheet lined with parchment paper (this cuts down on the grease and cleanup!). Bake at 375 degrees F for 8 to 10 minutes, or until the cookies are golden on the edges. If desired, sprinkle with a bit of natural sugar while the cookies are warm, and cool them on a cooling rack.

COOK'S TIP: These taste great dipped in low-fat milk or crumbled over frozen yogurt or ice cream.

Whole-Wheat Cornmeal Muffins

This is a tasty, high-fiber, low-fat muffin that can be eaten as a snack with a cup of low-fat milk or paired with some fresh fruit.

⅔ cup yellow cornmeal, degerminated
⅔ cup whole-wheat flour
1 tablespoon sugar
2 teaspoons baking powder
⅛ teaspoon salt
⅔ cup skim milk
2 egg whites
2 tablespoons canola oil

Total preparation and cooking time: 45 minutes

Makes 8 servings.

Nutrition information per serving:
Calories: 120
Fat: 4 g
  Saturated fat: 0 g
  Monounsaturated fat: 2 g
Cholesterol: 0 mg
Sodium: 180 mg
Carbohydrate: 19 g
Fiber: 2 g
Protein: 4 g

Preheat the oven to 400 degrees F. Grease 8 muffin tins, or use paper liners. Mix the dry ingredients thoroughly. Mix the milk, egg whites, and oil. Add these to the dry ingredients. Stir until the dry ingredients are barely moistened. The batter will be lumpy. Fill the muffin tins two-thirds full. Bake for about 20 minutes until lightly browned.

COOK'S TIP: To add some protein and a little crunch, include ½ ounce of walnuts to make this a protein-packed stand-alone snack that satisfies your hunger.

Brown Rice Pudding

This recipe, from my friend Cynthia's vegan kitchen, is creamy yet hearty and includes some of her favorite spices. The coconut and the star fruit are perfect complements in texture and sweetness, and Cynthia calls this "the ultimate comfort food."

½ cup instant brown rice
1 cup vanilla soy milk
⅛ teaspoon salt
⅛ teaspoon cinnamon
⅛ teaspoon nutmeg
2 tablespoons plump raisins
1 tablespoon egg replacer mixed with 1 tablespoon water
¼ teaspoon vanilla extract
2 tablespoons shredded coconut
1 tablespoon maple syrup
1 medium star fruit, sliced

Combine the rice, soy milk, salt, cinnamon, nutmeg, and raisins. Bring this to a rolling

Total preparation and cooking time: 20 minutes

Makes 2 servings.

Nutrition information per serving:
Calories: 350
Fat: 6 g
  Saturated fat: 3 g
  Monounsaturated fat: 1 g
Cholesterol: 0 mg
Sodium: 260 mg
Carbohydrate: 66 g
Fiber: 5 g
Protein: 9 g

boil, stirring constantly. Reduce the heat and simmer about 5 minutes, stirring less often until the rice fluffs. Mix the egg substitute with water. Slowly add this to the hot mixture, stirring until thick. Stir in the vanilla, coconut, and maple syrup. Divide the mixture into 2 pudding cups. Serve it warm or chilled. Top each with sliced star fruit just before serving.

COOK'S TIP: This is a dessert that eats like a meal and provides a good amount of fiber. It makes a tasty breakfast or, in a smaller portion, a great dessert.

APPENDIX A

Master Food Lists

The food lists in this appendix provide you with examples of how to fit your favorite foods and beverages into your individual meal plans. Along with the food lists provided in chapter 3, the following lists provide even more examples of what a portion looks like for many items you may choose in each food category emphasized in the Dietary Guidelines.

What Counts as 1 Cup of Fruit?

In general, 1 cup of fruit or of 100 percent fruit juice or ½ cup of dried fruit can be considered 1 cup from the fruit group. The following approximate amounts count as 1 cup of fruit (equivalents for ½ cup are also shown) toward your daily recommended intake:

Type of Fruit	1 Cup of Fruit Equals	½ Cup of Fruit Equals
Apple	½ large (3¼-inch diameter) 1 small (2½-inch diameter) 1 cup sliced or chopped, raw or cooked	½ cup sliced or chopped, raw or cooked
Applesauce	1 cup	1 snack container (4 oz.)
Banana	1 cup sliced 1 large (8 to 9 inches long)	1 small (less than 6 inches long)
Cantaloupe	1 cup diced or melon balls	1 medium wedge (⅛ medium melon)

(continued)

183

(continued)

	1 Cup of Fruit Equals	½ Cup of Fruit Equals
Dried fruit (raisins, prunes, apricots, etc.)	½ cup dried fruit = 1 cup fruit (e.g., ½ cup raisins, ½ cup prunes, ½ cup dried apricots)	¼ cup dried fruit = ½ cup fruit (1 small box of raisins, 1.5 oz.)
Grapes	1 cup whole or cut-up 32 seedless grapes	16 seedless grapes
Grapefruit	1 medium (4-inch diameter) 1 cup sections	½ medium (4-inch diameter)
Mixed fruit (fruit cocktail)	1 cup diced or sliced, raw or canned, drained	1 snack container (4 oz.), drained (⅜ cup)
100% fruit juice (orange, apple, grape, grapefruit, etc.)	1 cup	½ cup
Orange	1 large (3¹⁄₁₆-inch diameter) 1 cup sections	1 small (2⅜-inch diameter)
Orange, mandarin	1 cup canned, drained	½ cup, drained
Peach	1 large (2¾-inch diameter) 1 cup sliced or diced, raw, cooked, or canned, drained 2 halves, canned	1 small (2⅜-inch diameter), 1 snack container (4 oz), drained = ⅜ cup
Pear	1 medium pear (2½ per lb.) 1 cup sliced or diced, raw, cooked, or canned, drained	1 snack container (4 oz.), drained = ⅜ cup
Pineapple	1 cup chunks, sliced or crushed, raw, cooked or canned, drained	1 snack container (4 oz.), drained = ⅜ cup
Plum	1 cup sliced raw or cooked, 3 medium or 2 large plums	1 large plum
Strawberries	About 8 large berries, 1 cup whole, halved, or sliced, fresh or frozen	½ cup whole, halved, or sliced, fresh or frozen
Watermelon	1 small wedge (1-inch thick) 1 cup diced or balls	6 melon balls

What Counts as 1 Cup of Vegetables?

In general, 1 cup of raw or cooked vegetables or vegetable juice, or 2 cups of raw leafy greens can be considered 1 cup from the vegetable group. The table on pages 185–186 lists approximate amounts that count as 1 cup of vegetables (equivalents for ½ cup are also shown) toward your recommended intake.

	1 Cup of Vegetables Equals	½ Cup of Vegetables Equals
Dark Green Vegetables		

Broccoli	1 cup chopped or florets
	3 spears 5 inches long, raw
	  or cooked
		½ cup chopped or florets
		1½ spears 5 inches long,
		  raw or cooked

Greens (collards, mustard greens, turnip greens, kale)	1 cup cooked	½ cup cooked
Spinach	1 cup cooked 2 cups raw	1 cup raw
Raw leafy greens: spinach, romaine, watercress, dark green leafy lettuce, endive, escarole	2 cups raw	1 cup raw
Orange Vegetables		
Carrots	1 cup, strips, slices, or chopped, raw or cooked 2 medium carrots 1 cup baby carrots (12)	1 medium carrot 6 baby carrots
Pumpkin	1 cup mashed, cooked	½ cup mashed, cooked

Sweet potato	1 large baked (2½ inches
	  diameter)
	1 cup sliced, mashed, or
	  cooked
		½ large baked (2½ inches
		  diameter)
		½ cup sliced, mashed, or
		  cooked

Winter squash (acorn, butternut, or hubbard)	1 cup cubed, cooked	⅓ acorn squash, baked
Dry Beans and Peas		

Dry beans and peas (such
as black, garbanzo, kidney,
pinto, or soy beans, or
black-eyed peas or split peas
	1 cup whole or mashed,
	  cooked
		½ cup whole or mashed,
		  cooked

Tofu	1 cup ½-inch cubes (about
	  8 oz.)
		1 piece 2½-by-2¾-by-1
		  inches (about 4 oz.)

Starchy Vegetables		
Corn, yellow and white	1 cup kernels 1 large ear (8 to 9 inches long)	1 small ear (about 6 inches long)
Green peas	1 cup	½ cup

White potatoes	1 cup diced, mashed
	1 medium boiled or baked
	  potato (2½- to 3-inch
	  diameter)
	French fried: 20 medium to
	  long strips (2½ to 4 inches
	  long) (contains discretionary
	  calories and/or oils)
		½ cup diced, mashed
		French fried: 10 medium to
		  long strips (2½ to 4 inches
		  long) (contains discretionary
		  calories and/or oils)

(continued)

(continued)

	1 Cup of Vegetables Equals	½ Cup of Vegetables Equals
Other Vegetables		
Bean sprouts	1 cup cooked	½ cup cooked
Cabbage, green	1 cup chopped or shredded, raw or cooked	½ cup chopped or shredded, raw or cooked
Cauliflower	1 cup pieces or florets, raw or cooked	½ cup pieces or florets, raw or cooked
Celery	1 cup, diced or sliced, raw or cooked	½ cup diced or sliced, raw or cooked
	2 large stalks (11 to 12 inches long)	1 large stalk (11 to 12 inches long)
Cucumbers	1 cup raw, sliced or chopped	½ cup raw, sliced or chopped
Green or wax beans	1 cup cooked	½ cup cooked
Green or red peppers	1 cup chopped, raw or cooked	½ cup chopped, raw or cooked
	1 large pepper (3-inch diameter, 3¾ inches long)	1 small pepper
Lettuce, iceberg or head	2 cups raw, shredded or chopped	1 cup raw, shredded or chopped
Mushrooms	1 cup raw or cooked	½ cup raw or cooked
Onions	1 cup chopped, raw or cooked	½ cup chopped, raw or cooked
Tomatoes	1 large raw whole (3-inch)	1 small raw whole (2¼-inch)
	1 cup chopped or sliced, raw, canned, or cooked	½ cup chopped or sliced
		1 medium canned
Tomato or mixed vegetable juice	1 cup	½ cup
Summer squash or zucchini	1 cup cooked, sliced or diced	½ cup cooked, sliced or diced

What Counts as a 1-Ounce Equivalent of Grains?

In general, 1 slice of bread, 1 cup of ready-to-eat cereal, or ½ cup of cooked rice, cooked pasta, or cooked cereal can be considered a 1-ounce equivalent from the grains group. The table on page 187 lists approximate amounts that count as a 1-ounce equivalent of grains toward your daily recommended intake. In some cases, the number of ounce equivalents for common portions are also shown.

	1-oz. Equivalent Equals	Common Portions and Number of 1-oz. Equivalents They Count As
Bagels	½ mini bagel	1 large bagel = 4-oz. equivalents
Biscuits	1 small (2-inch diameter)	1 large (3-inch diameter) = 2-oz. equivalents
Breads (100% whole wheat Other grains: white, wheat, French, sourdough)	1 regular slice 1 small slice French 4 snack-size	2 regular slices = 2-oz. equivalents
Bulgur cracked wheat	½ cup cooked	
Cornbread	1 small piece (2½-by-1¼-by-1¼ inches)	1 medium piece (2½-by-2½-by-1¼ inches) = 2-oz. equivalents
Crackers (100% whole-wheat, rye, saltines, snack crackers)	5 whole-wheat crackers 2 rye crispbreads 7 square or round crackers	
English muffins	½ muffin	1 muffin = 2-oz. equivalents
Muffins (whole-wheat, bran, corn, plain)	1 small (2½-inch diameter)	1 large (3½-inch diameter) = 3-oz. equivalents
Oatmeal	½ cup cooked 1 packet instant 1 oz. dry (regular or quick)	
Pancakes (whole-wheat, buckwheat, buttermilk, plain)	1 pancake (4½-inch diameter) 2 small pancakes (3-inch diameter)	3 pancakes (4½-inch diameter) = 3-oz. equivalents
Pasta—spaghetti, macaroni, noodles	½ cup cooked 1 oz. dry	1 cup cooked = 2-oz. equivalents
Popcorn	3 cups, popped	1 microwave bag, popped = 4-oz. equivalents
Ready-to-eat breakfast cereal	1 cup flakes or rounds 1¼ cup puffed	
Rice (brown, wild, white)	½ cup cooked 1 oz. dry	1 cup cooked = 2-oz. equivalents
Tortillas	1 small flour tortilla (6-inch diameter) 1 corn tortilla (6-inch diameter)	1 large tortilla (12-inch diameter) = 4-oz. equivalents

What Counts as a 1-Ounce Equivalent in the Meat and Beans Group?

In general, 1 ounce of meat, poultry, or fish; ¼ cup cooked dry beans; 1 egg; 1 tablespoon of peanut butter; or ½ ounce of nuts or seeds can be considered a 1-ounce equivalent from the meat and beans group. The following table lists approximate amounts that count as 1-ounce equivalents in the meat and beans group toward your daily recommended intake. Common portions and the number of 1-ounce equivalents they equal are also given.

	1-oz. Equivalent Equals	Common Portions and Number of 1-oz. Equivalents It Counts As
Dry beans and peas	¼ cup of cooked dry beans (such as black, kidney, pinto, or white beans) ¼ cup of cooked dry peas (such as chickpeas, cowpeas, lentils, or split peas) ¼ cup of baked beans, refried beans ¼ cup (about 2 oz.) of tofu 1 oz. tempeh, cooked ¼ cup roasted soybeans 1 falafel patty (2¼-inch, 4 oz.) 2 tbsp. hummus	1 cup split pea soup = 2-oz. equivalents 1 cup lentil soup = 2-oz. equivalents 1 cup bean soup = 2-oz. equivalents 1 soy or bean burger patty = 2-oz. equivalents
Eggs	1 egg	
Fish	1 oz. cooked fish or shell fish	1 can of tuna, drained = 3- to 4-oz. equivalents 1 salmon steak = 4- to 6-oz. equivalents 1 small trout = 3-oz. equivalents
Meats	1 oz. cooked lean beef 1 oz. cooked lean pork or ham	1 small steak (eye of round, filet) = 3½- to 4-oz. equivalents 1 small lean hamburger = 2- to 3-oz. equivalent
Nuts and seeds	½ oz. of nuts (12 almonds, 24 pistachios, 7 walnut halves)[a] ½ oz. of seeds (pumpkin, sunflower, or squash seeds, hulled, roasted)[a] 1 tbsp. of peanut butter or almond butter[a]	1 oz. of nuts or seeds[b] = 2-oz. equivalents
Poultry	1 oz. cooked chicken or turkey, without skin 1 sandwich slice of turkey (4½-by-2½-by-⅛ inches)	1 small chicken breast half = 3-oz. equivalents ½ Cornish game hen = 4-oz. equivalents

[a]These also count as 1 teaspoon of oil.
[b]These also count as 2 teaspoons of oil.

What Counts as 1 Cup in the Milk Group?

The following table lists approximate amounts that count as 1 cup in the milk group toward your daily recommended intake.

	Amount That Counts as 1 Cup	Common Portions and the Number of Cups It Counts As
Cheese (low-fat or fat-free)	1½ oz. hard cheese (cheddar, mozzarella, Swiss, parmesan) ⅓ cup shredded cheese 2 oz. processed cheese (American) ½ cup ricotta cheese 2 cups cottage cheese	1 slice of hard cheese = ½ cup milk 1 slice of processed cheese = ⅓ cup milk ½ cup cottage cheese = ¼ cup milk
Milk-based desserts (fat-free or low-fat)	1 cup pudding made with milk 1 cup frozen yogurt 1½ cups ice cream	1 scoop ice cream = ⅓ cup milk
Skim milk	1 cup 1 half-pint container ½ cup evaporated milk	
Yogurt	1 regular container (8 fluid oz.) 1 cup	1 small container (6 oz.) = ¾ cup 1 snack-size container (4 oz.) = ½ cup

What Counts as 1 Teaspoon in the Oils Group?

The following table lists approximate amounts that count as 1 teaspoon of oil. Nuts, seeds, and nut butters, which naturally contain oils, are counted in the meat and beans group as well as the oils group. See page 188 for more on how to count nuts, seeds, and nut butters.

	Amount That Counts as 1 Teaspoon	Common Portions and the Approximate Number of Teaspoons They Count As
Avocado	⅛ small	½ small = 3 tsp.*
Black olives, large, pitted	8	4 = ½ tsp.
Black olives, small, pitted	15	7 = ½ tsp.
Green olives, queen size	7	3 = ½ tsp.
Green olives, stuffed	12	4 = ⅓ tsp.
Margarine, soft (trans fat–free)	1 tsp.	1 tbsp. = 3 tsp.

*Also counts as ½ cup fruit.

(continued)

(continued)

	Amount That Counts as 1 Teaspoon	Common Portions and the Approximate Number of Teaspoons They Count As
Margarine, soft (trans fat–free), light or low-fat	1 tbsp.	1 tbsp. = 1 tsp.
Mayonnaise	1 tsp.	1 tbsp. = 3 tsp.
Mayonnaise, light or low-fat	1 tbsp.	2 tbsp. = 2 tsp.
Mayonnaise-type salad dressing	1 tbsp.	2 tbsp. = 2 tsp.
Salad dressing (Italian)	1 tbsp.	2 tbsp. = 2 tsp.
Salad dressing, light or low-fat	2 tbsp.	2 tbsp. = 1 tsp.
Vegetable oils (such as canola, corn, cottonseed, olive, peanut, safflower, sesame, soybean, sunflower, walnut)	1 tsp.	1 tbsp. = 3 tsp.

How Do I Count the Solid Fats I Eat?

The following table gives a quick guide to the approximate amounts of solid fats added to or found in some common foods. All the calories listed count as discretionary calories.

	Amount of Food	Amount of Solid Fat in Teaspoons/Grams	Number of Discretionary Calories to Count As
Solid fats			
Butter	1 tbsp.	2½ tsp./12 g	100
Coconut oil or palm kernel oil	1 tbsp.	3 tsp./14 g	120
Margarine (hard or stick)	1 tbsp.	2½ tsp./11 g	100
Cream cheese	1 tbsp.	1 tsp./5 g	50
Foods made with solid fats			
Bacon, cooked	2 slices	1½ tsp./6 g	85
Biscuit	1 small (2½-inch diameter)	1½ tsp./6 g	125
Cheddar cheese	1½ oz.	3 tsp./14 g	170
Cheese danish	1 pastry (2½ oz.)	3½ tsp./16 g	265
Chocolate cream pie	⅙ of 8-inch pie	5 tsp./22 g	345

	Amount of Food	Amount of Solid Fat in Teaspoons/Grams	Number of Discretionary Calories to Count As
Foods made with solid fats			
Croissant	1 medium (2 oz.)	3 tsp./12 g	230
Half and half cream	1 tbsp.	½ tsp./2 g	20
Hamburger— regular (80% lean)	3 oz., cooked	3 tsp./14 g	205
Heavy cream	1 tbsp.	1 tsp./5 gr	50
Ice cream, chocolate	1 cup	3 tsp./14 g	285
Pork sausage	2 links (2 oz.)	3 tsp./14 g	165
Pound cake	¹⁄₁₂ of 12-ounce cake	1½ tsp./6 g	110
Prime rib roast, lean and fat (⅛-inch trim)	3 oz., cooked	6 tsp./29 g	340
Prime rib roast, lean only	3 oz., cooked	3½ tsp./16 g	250
Sour cream	1 tbsp.	½ tsp./2 g	25
Whole milk	1 cup	2 tsp./8 g	145

How Do I Count Mixed Meals (Meals That Contain Foods from More Than One Food Group)?

The following table shows how to count (approximately) some of the foods you may consume (especially when you eat out).

Food and Sample Portion Size	Counts As	Calories
Apple pie (1 slice)	2 grains, ¼ fruit	280
Bean and cheese burrito (1)	2½ grains, ⅛ vegetable, 1 milk, 2 meat and beans	445
Beef stir-fry (1 cup)	3/4 vegetable, 1½ meat and beans	165
Beef taco (2 tacos)	2½ grains, ¼ vegetable, ¼ milk, 2 meat and beans	370
Cheese pizza–thin crust (1 slice from medium pizza)	1 grain, ⅛ vegetable, ½ milk	215
Chef salad (3 cups, without dressing)	1½ vegetables, 3 meat and beans	230

(continued)

(*continued*)

Food and Sample Portion Size	Counts As	Calories
Chicken fried rice (1 cup)	1½ grains, ¼ vegetable, 1 meat and beans	270
Chicken pot pie (8-oz. pie)	2½ grains, ¼ milk, 1½ meats and beans	500
Clam chowder—Manhattan (chunky, 1 cup)	⅜ vegetable, 2 meats and beans	135
Clam chowder—New England (1 cup)	½ grain, ⅛ vegetable, ½ milk, 2 meats and beans	185
Cream of tomato soup (1 cup)	½ grain, ½ vegetable, ½ milk	160
Egg roll (1)	½ grain, ⅛ vegetable, ½ meat and beans	150
Large cheeseburger (3 oz. of meat)	2 grains, ⅓ milk, 3 meats and beans	500
Lasagna (1 piece 3½-by-4-inches)	2 grains, ½ vegetable, 1 milk, 1 meat	445
Macaroni and cheese (1 cup made from packaged mix)	2 grains, ½ milk	260
Pasta salad with vegetables (1 cup)	1½ grains, ½ vegetable	140
Peanut butter and jelly sandwich (1)	2 grains, 2 meats and beans, 2 oils	375
Pumpkin pie (1 slice)	1½ grains, ⅛ vegetable, ¼ milk, ¼ meat and beans	240
Stuffed peppers with rice and meat	½ grain, ½ vegetable, 1 meat and beans	190
Tuna noodle casserole (1 cup)	1½ grains, ½ milk, 2 meats and beans	260
Tuna salad sandwich	2 grains, ¼ vegetable, 2 meats and beans	290
Turkey sub (6 inches)	2 grains, ½ vegetable, ¼ milk, 2 meats and beans	320

APPENDIX B

Determining Your Calorie Needs

This appendix contains two other formulas that registered dietitians and other health professionals may use to help you estimate your calorie needs.

The Mifflin-St. Jeor Equation

This formula takes into account weight, height, age, and gender to calculate your resting metabolic rate (RMR) in kilocalories per day. Here's how you can estimate your daily calorie needs using the Mifflin-St. Jeor equation:

1. Convert your weight in pounds to kilograms: 1 kilogram = 2.2 pounds

2. Convert your height in inches to centimeters: 1 inch = 2.54 centimeters

3. Determine your RMR:
   Women: RMR = $(9.99 \times \text{weight}) + (6.25 \times \text{height}) - (4.92 \times \text{age}) - 161$
   Men: RMR = $(9.99 \times \text{weight}) + (6.25 \times \text{height}) - (4.92 \times \text{age}) + 5$

4. Multiply your RMR by the appropriate activity factor as follows:

- If you are sedentary (you do little or no exercise), multiply your RMR by 1.2.
- If you are lightly active (you do light exercise or sports 1 to 3 days per week), multiply your RMR by 1.375.
- If you are moderately active (you do moderate exercise or sports 3 to 5 days per week), multiply your RMR by 1.55.
- If you are very active (you do vigorous exercise or sports 6 to 7 days per week), multiply your RMR by 1.725.
- If you are extra active (you do vigorous daily exercise or sports and have a physical job or train twice a day), multiply your RMR by 1.9.

The Harris-Benedict Equation

This formula also takes into account height, weight, age, and gender to calculate your RMR. Here's how you can estimate your daily calorie needs using the Harris-Benedict equation:

1. Convert your weight in pounds to kilograms: 1 kilogram = 2.2 pounds

2. Convert your height in inches to centimeters: 1 inch = 2.54 centimeters

3. Determine your RMR:

    Women: RMR = 665.09 + (9.56 × weight in kilograms) + (1.84 × height in centimeters) − (4.67 × age in years).

    Men: RMR = 66.47 + (13.75 × weight in kilograms) + (5.0 × height in centimeters) − (6.75 × age in years)

4. Multiply your RMR by the appropriate activity factor as follows:

    - If you are sedentary (you do little or no exercise), multiply your RMR by 1.2.
    - If you are lightly active (you do light exercise or sports 1 to 3 days per week), multiply your RMR by 1.375.

- If you are moderately active (you do moderate exercise or sports 3 to 5 days per week), multiply your RMR by 1.55.
- If you are very active (you do vigorous exercise or sports 6 to 7 days per week), multiply your RMR by 1.725.
- If you are extra active (you do vigorous daily exercise or sports and have a physical job or train twice a day), multiply your RMR by 1.9.

Resources

Dietary Guidelines for Americans, **2005, 6th Edition**
United States Department of Health and Human Services (HHS)
and the United States Department of Agriculture (USDA)
www.healthierus.gov/dietaryguidelines

Dietary Guidelines for Americans Advisory Committee Report,
2005
www.health.gov/dietaryguidelines/dga2005/report

www.MyPyramid, the New Food Guidance System (USDA)
mypyramid.com

www.healthierus.gov
This Web site from HHS provides great information on nutrition
and physical fitness and provides links to a variety of government-
sponsored health Web sites.

www.foodsafety.gov
www.homefoodsafety.org
These Web sites provide great information about food safety.

www.americaonthemove.org
The America on the Move Foundation (AOMF), formerly the
Partnership to Promote Healthy Eating and Active Living, is a
national program that supports healthful eating and active living
habits in our society.

The AOMF recently launched the AOM Registry, which collects
data from individuals who successfully made and sustained lifestyle
changes.

www.nal.usda.gov/fnic/foodcomp
This Web site provides food composition data (for example, calo-
ries) for more than 7,300 foods that are available in the United
States.

win.niddk.nih.gov/index.htm
This Web site of the Weight Control Information Network (from HHS and NIH) provides great information on weight control, obesity, physical activity, and related nutritional issues.
1-800-WIN-8098

Centers for Disease Control and Prevention
www.cdc.gov

United States Department of Health and Human Services (HHS)
200 Independence Avenue, S.W.
Washington, DC 20201
202-619-0257
Toll free: 1-877-696-6775
www.hhs.gov

USDA Center for Nutrition Policy and Promotion
3101 Park Center Drive
Room 1034
Alexandria, VA 22302-1594
www.usda.gov/cnpp

United States Food and Drug Administration (FDA)
5600 Fishers Lane
Rockville, MD 20857-0001
1-888-INFO-FDA (1-888-463-6332)
www. FDA.gov
For information about the Nutrition Facts panels on food products, see www.cfsan.fda.gov/~dms/foodlab.html.
For information about Qualified Health Claims on food product labels, see www.cfsan.fda.gov/~dms/lab-qhc.html.

National Diabetes Information Clearinghouse
1 Information Way
Bethesda, MD 20892-3560
(301) 654-3327
Fax: (301) 907-8906
www.fda.gov/diabetes

National Heart, Lung, and Blood Institute
P.O. Box 30105
Bethesda, MD 20824-0105
(301) 251-1222
Fax: (301) 251-1223
www.nhlbi.nih.gov

National Institute of Diabetes and Digestive and Kidney Diseases
31 Center Drive, MSC-2560
Building 31, Room 9A-04
Bethesda, MD 20892-2560
(301) 496-3583
Fax: (301) 496-7422
www.niddk.nih.gov

Professional Organizations

American Cancer Society
Atlanta, Georgia
1-800-ACS-2345
www.cancer.org

American College of Sports Medicine
P.O. Box 1440
Indianapolis, IN 46206-1440
(317) 637-9200
Fax: (317) 634-7817
www.acsm.org

American Diabetes Association
National Call Center
1701 North Beauregard Street
Alexandria, VA 22311
1-800 DIABETES (1-800-342-2383)
Fax: 815-734-1223
www.diabetes.org
askADA@diabetes.org

American Dietetic Association
120 S. Riverside Plaza, Suite 2000
Chicago, IL 60606-6995
(800) 877-1600
Fax: (312) 899-1979
www.eatright.org
To find a registered dietitian in your area, call 1-800-366-1655.

Center for Science in the Public Interest (CSPI)
Publishes *Nutrition Action Health Letter*.
1875 Connecticut Ave, NW Suite 300
Washington, DC 20009-5728
202-332-9110
Fax: 202-265-4954
www.cspinet.org

National Cancer Institute
Office of Cancer Communications
9000 Rockville Pike
Building 31, Room 10A-24
Bethesda, MD 20892
(800) 4-CANCER (800-422-6237)
www.nci.nih.gov

North American Association for the Study of Obesity (NAASO)
8630 Fenton Street, Suite 918
Silver Spring, MD 20910
(301) 563-6526
Fax: (301) 587-6595
www.nasso.org

Other Resources

Ruth Winter, M.S. *A Consumer's Dictionary of Food Additives, 6th Edition*. Three Rivers Press, 2004.

Environmental Nutrition: The Newsletter of Food, Nutrition and Health
P.O. Box 5656
Norwalk, CT 06856-5656
Customer_Service@belvoir.com
800-424-7887
Fax: 203-857-3103
www.environmentalnutrition.com

sowhatcanieat.com
Visit Elisa Zied at sowhatcanieat.com and elisazied.com to learn more about the author and to subscribe to a free newsletter that features tips and recipes to help you incorporate the Dietary Guidelines into your life.

References

Bazzano, L. A., M. K. Serdula, and S. Liu. 2003. Dietary intake of fruits and vegetables and risk of cardiovascular disease. *Current Atherosclerosis Reports* 5:492–9.

Centers for Disease Control and Prevention Primary Prevention Working Group. 2004. Primary prevention of type 2 diabetes mellitus by lifestyle intervention: implications for health policy. *Annals of Internal Medicine* 140:951–7.

Davidson, T. L., and S. E. Swithers. 2004. A Pavlovian approach to the problem of obesity. *International Journal of Obesity and Related Metabolic Disorders* 28:933–5.

Dietary Reference Intakes for Energy, Carbohydrate, Fiber, Fat, Fatty Acids, Cholesterol, Protein, and Amino Acids (prepublication version). Panel on Macronutrients, Panel on the Definition of Dietary Fiber, Subcommittee on Upper Reference Levels of Nutrients, Subcommittee on Interpretation and Uses of Dietary Reference Intakes, and the Standing Committee on the Scientific Evaluation of Dietary Reference Intakes. Institute of Medicine of the National Academies, the National Academies Press, Washington, DC, 2002.

Duyff, R. L. 2002. *American Dietetic Association Complete Food and Nutrition Guide*, 2nd ed. Hoboken, NJ: John Wiley & Sons, Inc.

Frankenfield, D., L. Roth-Yousey, and C. Compher. 2005. Comparison of predictive equations for resting metabolic rate in healthy nonobese and obese adults: a systematic review. *Journal of the American Dietetic Association* 105:775–89.

Harris, J. A., and F. G. Benedict. 1919. *A Biometric Study of Basal Metabolism in Man.* Publication no. 279. Washington, DC: Carnegie Institute of Washington.

Hung, H. C., K. J. Joshipura, R. Jiang, F.B. Hu, D. Hunter, S. A. Smith-Warner, G. A. Colditz, B. Rosner, D. Spiegelman, and W. C. Willet. 2004. Fruit and vegetable intake and risk of major chronic disease. *Journal of the National Cancer Institute* 96:1577–84.

Insel, P., R. E. Turner, and D. Ross. 2004. *Nutrition*, 2nd ed. Sudbury, MA: Jones and Bartlett Publishers.

Jensen, M. K., P. Koh-Banerjee, F. B. Hu, M. Franz, L. Sampson, M. Gronbaek, and E. B. Rimm. 2004. Intakes of whole grains, bran, and germ and the risk of coronary heart disease in men. *American Journal of Clinical Nutrition* 80:1492–9.

Joint WHO/FAO Expert Consultation on Diet, Nutrition, and the Prevention of Chronic Diseases (2002: Geneva, Switzerland). *Diet, Nutrition and the Prevention of Chronic Diseases: report of a joint WHO/FAO Expert Consultation*, 2003.

Kalkwarf, H. J., J. C. Khoury, and B. P. Lanphear. 2003. Milk intake during childhood and adolescence, adult bone density, and osteoporotic fractures in U.S. women. *American Journal of Clinical Nutrition* 77:257–65.

Koh-Banerjee, P., M. Franz, L. Sampson, S. Liu, D. R. Jacobs Jr., D. Spiegelman, W. Willett, and E. Rimm. 2004. Changes in wholegrain, bran, and cereal fiber consumption in relation to 8-y weight gain among men. *American Journal of Clinical Nutrition* 80:1237–45.

Liu, S., W. C. Willett, J.E. Manson, F. B. Hu, B. Rosner, and G. Colditz. 2003. Relation between changes in intakes of dietary fiber and grain products and changes in weight and development of obesity among middle-aged women. *American Journal of Clinical Nutrition* 78:920–7.

Mifflin, M. D., S. T. St. Jeor, L.A. Hill, B. J. Scott, S. A. Daugherty, and Y.O. Koh. 1990. A new predictive equation for resting energy expenditure in healthy individuals. *American Journal of Clinical Nutrition* 51:241–7.

Moore, L. L., A. J. Visioni, M. M. Qureshi, M. L. Bradlee, R. C. Ellison, and R. D'Agostino. 2005. Weight loss in overweight adults and the long-term risk of hypertension: the Framingham study. *Archives in Internal Medicine* 165:1298–1303.

Pereira, M. A., A. I. Kartashov, C. B. Ebbeling, L. Van Horn, M. L. Slattery, D. R. Jacobs Jr., and D. S. Ludwig. 2005. Fast-food habits, weight gain, and insulin resistance (the CARDIA study): 15-year prospective analysis. *Lancet* 365:36–42.

Rolls, B., L. S. Roe, and J. S. Meengs. 2004. Salad and satiety: Energy density and portion size of a first-course salad affect energy intake at lunch. *Journal of the American Dietetic Association* 104:1570–6.

Slavin, J. L. 2005. Dietary Fiber and Body Weight. *Nutrition* 21(3):411–8.

Tohill, B. C., J. Seymour, M. Serdula, L. Kettel-Khan, and B. J. Rolls. 2004. What epidemiologic studies tell us about the relationship between fruit and vegetable consumption and body weight. *Nutrition Reviews* 62:365–74.

Wu, X., G. R. Beecher, J. M. Holden, D. B. Haytowita, S. E. Gebhardt, and R. L. Prior. 2004. Lipophilic and hydrophilic antioxidant capacities of common foods in the United States. *Journal of Agricultural and Food Chemistry* 52:4026–37.

Index

Page numbers in italics refer to tables.